SECOND EDITION

REAL-TIME ULTRASOUND

A Manual for Physicians and Technical Personnel

ROYAL J. BARTRUM, JR., M.D.

HARTE C. CROW, M.D.

Department of Diagnostic Radiology
Dartmouth–Hitchcock
Medical Center
Hanover, New Hampshire

W.B. SAUNDERS COMPANY

1983   Philadelphia   London   Toronto   Mexico City   Rio de Janeiro   Sydney   Tokyo

W. B. Saunders Company: West Washington Square
                            Philadelphia, PA   19105

                            1 St. Anne's Road
                            Eastbourne, East Sussex BN21 3UN, England

                            1 Goldthorne Avenue
                            Toronto, Ontario M8Z 5T9, Canada

                            Apartado 26370—Cedro 512
                            Mexico 4, D.F., Mexico

                            Rua Coronel Cabrita, 8
                            Sao Cristovao Caixa Postal 21176
                            Rio de Janeiro, Brazil

                            9 Waltham Street
                            Artarmon, N.S.W. 2064, Australia

                            Ichibancho, Central Bldg., 22-1 Ichibancho
                            Chiyoda-Ku, Tokyo 102, Japan

Library of Congress Cataloging in Publication Data

Bartrum, Royal J.

Real-time ultrasound.

Rev. ed. of: Gray-scale ultrasound. 1977.

Bibliography: p.

Includes index,

1. Diagnosis, Ultrasonic—Handbooks, manuals, etc.
   I. Crow, Harte C.   II. Title. [DNLM: 1. Ultrasonics—
   Diagnostic use. WB 289 B294r]

RC78.7.U4B36 1983   616.07'543   82–47765

ISBN 0–7215–1552–X   AACR2

Real-Time Ultrasound:
A Manual for Physicians and Technical Personnel   ISBN   0-7216-1552-X

Last digit is the print number: 9   8   7   6   5   4   3   2   1

To Jane and Ann, who continue to support us with good counsel, encouragement, and patience.

PREFACE TO THE SECOND EDITION

In the preface to the first edition of this book we spent some time documenting the evolution of ultrasound in the United States and establishing the need for an introductory text. In the mid 1970's there were still a few skeptics who felt that ultrasound was a will-of-the-wisp that would soon be diffused by the emergence of modern CT scanners. The skeptics were both right and wrong. They were correct in their predictions of rapid evolution and progress for CT scanners; however, they were incorrect in predicting the demise of ultrasound. Not only has ultrasound survived, it is used in virtually every medical community in the country and is considered a staple of modern diagnostic imaging.

The secret to the durability of ultrasound scanning has been its continued technologic development and innovation. In the preface to the first edition we chronicled the amazing pace of development in the early 1970's; during this time scanners evolved from primitive bi-stable instruments, the pictures from which looked more like satellite weather maps than human anatomy, to gray-scale scanners that produced readily recognizable images of internal organs. This developmental pace has not abated; if anything, it has accelerated. The gray-scale scanner that was state-of-the-art in 1977 is a relic in 1982; in retrospect, it seems amazing that anyone could have gotten so much information from those machines!

While this continuing advancement in the field was exciting and satisfying, for us it had a serious drawback. The first edition of our manual became obsolete along with the equipment and scanning techniques it described. When it became apparent to us that our scanning techniques had undergone practically a 100 per cent revision, we concluded that a second edition was necessary.

The purpose of the second edition remains the same as that of the first with only minor modifications. Our goal is to provide an introduction to ultrasound (excluding echocardiology) to those who are new to the field and plan to work in the area. We hope that having read this text, the nascent ultrasonographer will be prepared to begin scanning and making diagnoses. As with the first edition, we have tried to keep medical and technical jargon to a minimum and stress the practical and easily understood approaches to scanning. Although the goals remain unchanged, the content has not. The second edition is more than 90 per cent rewritten, a reflection of the extensive changes that have occurred in the past five years.

The most obvious difference is the title. The first edition was entitled *Gray-Scale Ultrasound: A Manual for Physicians and Technical Personnel* to stress the important technologic innovation of the period, the introduction of gray-scale scanners. The title for the second edition has been changed to acknowledge the major technologic innovation of the early 1980's, the high-resolution real-time scanner. We have eliminated some chapters that are now obsolete. The former edition's chapter on laboratory organization has been deleted because it is unlikely that many new facilities are being set up in 1982. The use of ultrasonically guided percutaneous biopsy is now so widespread as to no longer justify an entire chapter. Bi-stable scanners have passed from the scene, and so has the chapter on this scanning technique. The chapters on clinical examinations have been expanded to include not only scanning techniques but established diagnostic criteria. Recent new uses of ultrasound such as the examination of the extracranial carotid arteries and neonatal brain have been included.

One thing that we hope has not changed is the writing style and the acceptance of the text. The first edition was considered somewhat "radical" in that the writing style did not conform to conventional medical textbooks. We felt at the time that there was a need for a less formal type of medical text on the subject, and the wide acceptance of this style has been gratifying. We hope that you will read this book in the spirit in which it was written; not as an encyclopedic catalog of diagnostic ultrasound, but as the attempt of two ultrasonographers to convey, in a useful way, their experiences in this rapidly changing and exciting field.

ROYAL J. BARTRUM, JR.
HARTE C. CROW

ACKNOWLEDGMENTS

Any book is like an iceberg: the authors are the tip, and supporting them is a large group of unseen collaborators. We would like to thank the following people who made this book possible. Good ultrasound is the product of close collaboration between technical personnel and physician. This book is based largely on the work of three sonographers, Sheila Foote, Carol Bailey, and Elizabeth LaBombard — whose skill and professionalism serve as inspiration for us all. Without their continuous support, none of this would have been possible. Our colleagues in the Radiology Department at the Dartmouth-Hitchcock Medical Center have been most supportive when our attention to ultrasound has called us away from other radiologic duties. Terri Soule, Vera Nichols, and Janet Wilson have shown uncommon patience at translating our hieroglyphic scrawls and retyping our perpetually revised manuscripts. Finally, our patients deserve special mention. They provide the ultimate source of our knowledge about the ultrasonic appearance of disease, and it is to their benefit that we direct our diagnostic efforts.

CONTENTS

Chapter 1

PRACTICAL PHYSICS

Do not skip this chapter! We hate physics just as much as you do, probably more. It would be wonderful if ultrasound scanners were totally standardized and automated so that all that was required to produce an image was simply to place the patient in front of the machine, push a button, and develop a picture. Alas, this is not the case at the present time. There is no field of medical imaging that is more dependent upon the skill of the machine operator than ultrasound scanning. And it is impossible to become a competent machine operator unless you know something about how the machine works.

We do not mean that you have to know enough physics to tear the scanner apart and rebuild the insides with leftover color TV parts, bubble gum, and a bobby pin; or that you have to be able to crystallize your own transducers on the kitchen stove. We mean that you must have a basic understanding of what the ultrasound beam is, why an echo is produced, why artifacts exist, and what the various knobs on the machine do to the picture and why.

This is similar to the knowledge you must have to operate any mechanical contrivance adequately. The automobile is a good example. Most of us are not mechanics and don't know a piston from a pushrod or preignition from a marble in the ashtray, yet we do know a fair amount about the practical physics of the car. For instance, we know that gasoline is burned in the engine and produces energy to run the rest of the car. We know that this process is started by another form of energy, electricity in the battery, which runs the starter. Therefore if we turn the key and nothing happens we are more likely to suspect that the battery is dead than that the car is out of gas. Knowing this, we would ask someone to give us a push start rather than setting off down the road, gas can in hand. Similarly if we were driving along and the car stopped, we would think the problem was more likely to be an empty gas tank than a dead battery.

It is this same general level of knowledge of the practical physics of ultrasound image pro-duction that is required. That is what this chapter is about—the physics of ultrasound for those who hate physics. We wish we could have put it at the end of the book—we know it is a bummer and a terrible lead-off topic—but unfortunately it is the basic platform upon which all ultrasound scanning rests, and you simply must understand some of it before any other aspect of scanning will make much sense.

Enough procrastination. Getting into physics is like getting into an ice-cold swimming pool; the only way to do it is to hold your nose and jump.

THE PULSE-ECHO PRINCIPLE

Ultrasonography is based on the pulse-echo principle. A man stands on one side of a canyon and shouts "Hello!" toward the other side. This is the "pulse." That pulse travels through the air at the speed of sound (about 741 miles an hour) until it hits the opposite wall of the canyon, where it is reflected back toward the man. Once the pulse has been reflected it becomes an "echo." The echo travels back to the man at the same speed of sound, and after a short time, he hears the echo. We have all participated in this type of pulse-echo experience.

If the man has a stopwatch (and a small electronic calculator) he can use this pulse and echo to calculate how far it is to the other side of the canyon. He simply measures the time it took for his shout (the pulse) to be echoed back to him. Suppose this was 4 seconds. He consults his handy conversion table, which tells him that 741 miles per hour is equivalent to 1087 feet per second. He then multiplies 1087 feet per second by 4 seconds and discovers that his "Hello" traveled 4348 feet. Since this repre-sented two trips across the canyon (one for the pulse going and the other for the echo return-ing) he then divides by 2 and obtains 2174 feet as the distance to the other side of the canyon.

Now if the man got a kick out of measuring canyons this way, he would probably get tired of doing all these calculations every time he shouted. Instead he would sit down with a six-pack and do all the calculations once for every possible time from 1 to, say, 20 seconds. He would then repaint the face of his stopwatch so that, instead of reading in seconds, it would read in the number of feet to the echo source. Then he would be all set to measure canyons easily and quickly, using only his shout and the calibrated watch. Of course, his calibrated watch would be accurate only as long as the speed of sound was 1087 feet per second, but since the speed of sound in air doesn't vary much, at least when compared with the accuracy with which he can read his stopwatch, this problem isn't of much concern.

ULTRASOUND

Ultrasound imaging uses this same pulse-echo principle. A short pulse of ultrasound is discharged into the body. This pulse travels through the tissues at a constant speed until it encounters a reflecting surface. At such a surface some of the sound beam is reflected back toward the source; there it is received by the ultrasound scanner, which has been keeping track of the time and converting it to a distance in the same manner as the man and his calibrated stopwatch. Instead of giving out the distance as a number, however, the scanner shows it as a dot or a spike on an oscilloscope or video screen; the position of the spike is proportional to the distance the echo traveled. This enables us not only to measure the distance but to get a visual picture of it as well.

Although the principle of ultrasonic pulse-echo diagnosis is the same as that of the echo in the canyon, there are several practical differences. To understand these differences we need to know a little about sound.

All sound, be it ultrasound or the kind we hear, is actually a series of repeating pressure waves. It is convenient to think about these waves and illustrate them as sine wave forms, as shown in Figure 1-1. Line A shows a single wave or cycle. As we move along the horizontal axis, which represents time, the pressure starts at zero, rises to a peak, then falls back to zero and continues to a negative value before returning to zero. Line B shows a continuous wave form in which a large number of the single waves have been strung together. The single wave is analogous to an extremely short beep of a car horn, while the continuous wave represents the horn being stuck in the on position.

Examsmanship department: Physicists use several terms to describe the way a wave is propagated in tissue; these are of no importance in clinical ultrasound but for obscure reasons seem to turn up on examinations. If ever asked you should say that ultrasound uses *longitudinal* or *compression* waves, not *shear* or *transverse* waves.

This simple wave form is not adequate to describe the sound fully, however. We must know more about the wave before we can predict how it will behave. Therefore, several pieces of information are described for these waves (such data are called parameters of the wave). Some of the more important parameters are illustrated in Figure 1-2. The **period** is the time it takes to complete a single cycle (about 0.3 of a microsecond for a typical wave). The **amplitude** is the peak pressure or height of the wave. This is a measure of the strength or "loudness" of the sound wave. A shouted "Hello" has a large amplitude, while a whispered "Hello" has a small amplitude. We will use the words *power, intensity,* and *loudness* interchangeably with *amplitude.* While, in a strict physical sense, each of these terms has a slightly different meaning, for our purposes it will cause no errors to think of them as describing the same quantity. The only time it is important to make the distinction between them is when discussing bioeffects and patient exposure.

The **velocity** is the speed of the wave. The velocity depends on the type and temperature

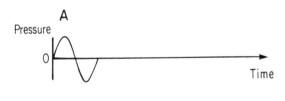

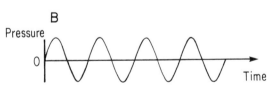

Figure 1-1. A diagrammatic representation of sound as a sine wave.

A. A single wave or cycle. The horizontal axis is time; the vertical axis is pressure at a point in the medium through which the sound is traveling. The wave starts at zero pressure, rises to a positive value, then falls past zero to a negative value before returning to its starting position.

B. A continuous sound wave made up of several single cycles linked together.

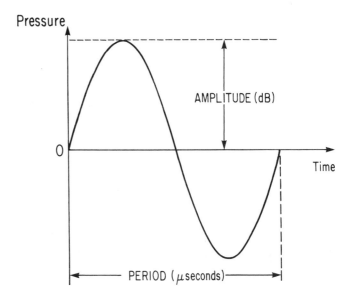

VELOCITY (meters/sec) = Speed of sound (~1540 meters/second for human soft tissue)

FREQUENCY (MHz) = 1/PERIOD

WAVELENGTH (millimeters) = VELOCITY / FREQUENCY

Figure 1–2. Some of the common parameters of a sound beam and the units in which they are commonly expressed.

of the material in which the wave is traveling; the denser the material, the greater the speed. For instance, in air sound travels 741 miles per hour, which is equivalent to 331 meters per second (from here on we will use the metric system for all measurements). In the much denser stainless steel, sound travels at 3100 meters per second. And in the intermediate density of human soft tissue at 37° C (body temperature), sound travels at 1540 meters per second. The difference in density between the various soft tissue organs of the body (e.g., liver, kidneys, pancreas, uterus) is very small, as is the variation in body temperature; therefore we can consider the speed of ultrasound in the living body to be constant—1540 meters per second.

The **frequency** is the number of times the wave is repeated per second. The frequency is calculated by dividing the period (the time it takes to complete a single cycle) into 1.

Finally there is the **wavelength,** which is the distance the wave travels during a single cycle. The wavelength is calculated by dividing the velocity by the frequency.

Fortunately we will not have to be concerned with making all these calculations, since only a very few different frequencies and wavelengths are used in ultrasound and it is easy to remember them.

Now we can see how ultrasound differs from the sound we hear. First, and most important, is frequency. Audible sound ranges in frequency from 16 to 20,000 cycles per second (a cycle per second is known as a hertz, abbreviated Hz; a million cycles per second is called a megahertz and is abbreviated MHz). Ultrasound is defined as any sound with a frequency greater than 20,000 Hz. In abdominal scanning we use sound frequencies ranging from 1 to 10 MHz.

The next consideration is velocity. Since we hear sound in air, the velocity of audible sound is 331 meters per second. We use ultrasound in human soft tissue, however, so the velocity in which we are interested is 1540 meters per second.

The wavelengths of audible sound range from 2 to 2000 centimeters (cm), while the wavelengths used in ultrasound are much shorter, from 0.1 to 1.5 millimeters (mm). (A millimeter is one tenth of a centimeter; a Virginia Slims cigarette is 120 mm long.)

The amplitude or power of the ultrasound used for diagnosis is much smaller than that needed to shout "Hello." Since amplitudes vary so widely, and since, for most purposes, we are not as concerned with the actual amplitude as with the relationship of one amplitude to another, a different type of measure of amplitude is used for sound. This is the decibel (dB) notation, which is based on comparing the amplitudes of two different sound waves. We are all familiar with this type of measurement and use it every day. For example, in describing the virtues of a football quarterback we might say that quarterback A can throw the ball twice as far as quarterback B can; or we say that a Mack truck weighs 10 times as much as a Volkswagen. In neither case do we talk about the actual number of feet the football is thrown or the number of pounds the truck weighs. Of course, if we have in our mind some concept of how much a Volkswagen weighs (perhaps from tipping one over in our younger days) we could describe other vehicles in terms of how they compare with a Volkswagen and, at the same time, have some idea of their actual weight as well. In this sense a comparative measurement system can be used as if the numbers corresponded to some real quantity. Even though it is not really correct to use decibels as if they were a real and absolute measure of sound amplitude or power, it is useful and convenient to do so and will not introduce any errors into our thinking. So, we will often refer to the amplitude of ultrasound echoes as X number of decibels; the greater the number of decibels, the greater the amplitude of (or the "louder") the echo.

Before we leave this topic of decibels, we should point out that this is a logarithmic system; that is, a decibel is defined as:

$$dB = 20 \log \frac{E_2}{E_1} ;$$

where E_2 and E_1 are the actual measurements of the amplitudes of two different echoes.* Logarithmic scales are used whenever the quantities involved cover very large ranges; this enables widely different numbers to be compared easily. You have probably noticed already that 20 dB corresponds to a factor of 10. Thus if echo A is 20 dB louder than echo B, echo A has 10 times the amplitude of echo B.

$$\log \frac{A}{B} = \log \frac{10}{1} = 1; 20 \log \frac{10}{1} = 20$$

---

*This definition of the decibel is used when electric power is involved, and since echoes produce electric signals, this is the definition used in diagnostic ultrasound. For other purposes the decibel is defined as:

$$dB = 10 \log \frac{P_2}{P_1}.$$

In a typical abdominal or pelvic ultrasound scan the echoes received from the soft tissues range in strength from 0 to 100 dB. The actual amplitude range of these echoes is therefore 1 to 1,000,000. (You probably have also figured out that quarterback A is 6 dB better than quarterback B and that a Mack truck is 20 dB heavier than a Volkswagen.)

INTERACTION OF ULTRASOUND AND TISSUE

Sound traveling through air, such as the "Hello" of our friend the canyon measurer, has a pretty uncomplicated life. It simply zips across the canyon, hits the far wall, and comes rebounding back. About the only really noticeable change is that the sound gets weaker as it travels, so the echo is not nearly as loud as the shout. When an ultrasonic pulse is sent into the soft tissues of the body, however, it undergoes continuous modification.

The most significant change is **attenuation**. Although this is not a scientifically rigorous definition, we shall consider attenuation to be the progressive weakening of the sound beam as it travels through tissue. Thus, the farther through the tissue the sound travels, the weaker it gets. The attenuation of ultrasound is dependent on many factors, including the wavelength of the sound, the type and density of the tissue, the degree of heterogeneity of the tissue, and the number and type of echo interfaces in the tissue. It is impossible to predict accurately the degree of attenuation for something as complex as human tissue. Nevertheless, it is no great problem to measure the attenuation in a laboratory (the amplitude of the sound beam is measured at varying distances in a tissue, and the difference, after some mathematical manipulation, becomes the attenuation).

Attenuation measurements have been made for many different human tissues with many different frequencies of ultrasound. These figures are available in textbooks on the physics of ultrasound. The actual numbers are of no great concern to the average clinical ultrasonographer, but it is useful to remember the following general rule of thumb: the "average" attenuation of an ultrasound beam in human soft tissue is 1 dB per centimeter per megahertz. This means that an ultrasound beam with a frequency of 1 MHz loses 1 dB of amplitude for every centimeter it travels. A 2.25 MHz beam loses $2.25 \times 1 = 2.25$ dB for every centimeter it travels, and a 5 MHz beam loses

5 × 1 = 5 dB per centimeter. We must remember that each echo received has actually traveled twice as far as the distance to the reflecting surface, since it has made a trip to the reflecting surface and back to the source. Therefore, we must multiply the attenuation by 2 if we wish to know how much an echo from any given depth has been attenuated.

Short quiz: Just to make sure we all have this straight before going on. *The question:* An ultrasound beam with a frequency of 3.5 MHz is directed into the liver, and an echo is received from a depth of 6 cm. How much has this echo been attenuated? *The answer:* Attenuation is estimated as 1 dB per centimeter per megahertz; 1 dB × 3.5 MHz = 3.5 dB per centimeter. This number is called the "attenuation coefficient." The echo came from 6 cm, but it actually traveled 12 cm—6 going out and 6 coming back—so we multiply 3.5 dB per centimeter by 12 cm and get 42 dB. The echo was attenuated by 42 dB.

How does attenuation of an ultrasound beam occur? Primarily through three processes: absorption, reflection, and scattering.

Absorption occurs when energy in the sound beam is captured (or absorbed) by the tissue. Most of this energy is converted to heat in the tissue. It is this process that is the basis for ultrasound diathermy, a common therapeutic use of ultrasound. At the low energy levels used in diagnostic ultrasound, the biologic effect of absorption is negligible, however.

Reflection is the redirection of a portion of the ultrasound beam back toward its source. Reflection gives rise to echoes and forms the basis of diagnostic ultrasound scanning. Whenever the sound beam passes from a tissue of one acoustic impedance to a tissue of a different acoustic impedance, a small portion of the beam will be reflected and the remainder will continue on. We shall take a closer look at this process in a minute.

Scattering occurs when the beam encounters an interface that is irregular and smaller than the sound beam. As the name suggests, the portion of the beam that interacts with this interface is "scattered" in all directions. This is similar to what happens to a cream pie when it is thrown in a face—the cream is splattered in many directions. There is no reason for the clinical ultrasonographer to know much about scattering other than that it occurs. Since the interfaces that produce scattering are small, only a small percentage of the beam is involved. (The portion of the beam that is "scattered" directly backward will return to the transducer and produce an echo—known as a non-specular reflection.)

There are two other closely related phenomena, **refraction** and **diffraction**, which are often (incorrectly) listed as causes of ultrasound attenuation. These terms refer to the bending of the sound beam as it crosses areas with differing tissue density. Although bending the beam does not cause it to be attenuated, it does decrease the amplitude of the returning echoes and produces the same effect as attenuation. Refraction is a common cause of artifacts, and we shall look at this process in some detail in Chapter 4.

REFLECTION AND ECHO PRODUCTION

We need to examine the process of ultrasonic reflection and echo production in a little detail, since it is the basis of scanning. Also there seems to be a great deal of confusion and misconception concerning this phenomenon, particularly in regard to the "resolution" of ultrasound systems.

Reflection occurs—that is, an echo is produced—whenever the ultrasound beam passes from a tissue of one acoustic impedance to a tissue of a different acoustic impedance. This is also known as crossing an acoustic impedance mismatch or as crossing an acoustic interface. The large number of terms used to describe this probably helps to account for the confusion. We will refer to this as an acoustic interface or simply an interface. An **interface** occurs whenever two tissues of differing acoustic impedance are in contact with each other.

Now all we need to know is what is "acoustic impedance"? Elementary, my dear Watson. The **acoustic impedance** of a tissue is the product of the density of the tissue and the speed of sound in the tissue. This is often written as: $Z = \rho \times c$, where Z = the acoustic impedance, ρ = the density of the tissue, and c = the speed of sound in the tissue. But the speed of sound in soft tissues is assumed to be a constant (1540 meters per second), so the only thing that affects the acoustic impedance is the density of the tissue. This simplifies matters greatly. For our purposes we can assume that the acoustic impedance is the same thing as the density of a tissue; therefore, an interface occurs every time tissues of different density are in contact with each other. It takes only very small density differences to make an interface: Water, blood cells, fat, liver cells, bile, bile duct walls, blood vessel walls, and connective or fibrous tissue all have sufficiently differing densities to create interfaces. This is one of the reasons ultrasound has proved so useful in abdominal and pelvic examinations; there is a tremendous amount of information about the soft tissues in the ultrasound beam. (Conventional x-rays, by contrast, cannot differentiate these small differences in density; blood cells, liver cells, bile, bile ducts, blood vessels, and connective and fibrous tissue all appear gray to the x-ray. CT scanners can inprove on ordinary x-rays by distinguishing smaller density differences, but even CT falls short of ultrasound.)

When the sound beam crosses an interface, only a small percentage of it is reflected. The remainder continues on through the tissues, where it can be reflected by other interfaces. The amount of sound that is reflected at an interface determines how much amplitude the returning echo will have or how "loud" the echo will be. This amount depends on how great the difference is between the two acoustic impedances that make up the interface. If the difference is very small, only a small percentage of the sound will be reflected; if the difference is large, a large portion will be reflected.

It would seem logical that large echoes would be desirable, but actually this is not the case. Ideally only enough of the beam should be reflected to enable the echo to be detected by the scanner; we want the rest of it to be available for creating other echoes. If too large a portion of the beam is reflected at an interface (producing a very loud echo), there is too little of the sound left to produce echoes from other interfaces deeper in the tissue. This is why ultrasound scanners cannot "see" through bowel gas or bone. The difference in acoustic impedance between soft tissue and gas or bone is very large, so large in fact that most of the beam is reflected and none is left to continue deeper. For example, at a soft tissue–bone interface about 70 per cent of the beam is reflected. It takes only two interfaces like this to exhaust the sound. For a soft tissue–gas interface the percentage is over 99 per cent. We can see that bone and gas are the ultrasonic equivalent of a stone wall; nothing gets through them. We should also notice that we are talking about percentage reflection. No matter how powerful the ultrasound beam, the same percentage will be reflected. If we use a louder beam we will get a louder echo but we won't penetrate the gas or bone. It's the same situation as shining a light at a mirror—no matter how bright the light, you cannot see through the mirror; you

just get a lot of glare. This is important because many people seem to believe that they can blast the sound beam through bowel gas by turning up the power. Although turning up the power makes more echoes, these echoes are mostly artifacts and have no relation to the underlying tissue. Because the problem of artifacts is so great we shall discuss it in greater detail in Chapter 4.

Extra reading for aggressive students department: Why are the acoustic impedances of soft tissue and gas or bone so different? You'll remember that acoustic impedance, Z, is actually the product of density and speed of sound. For soft tissues the speed of sound is nearly constant, so only the density factor is involved in changing the value of Z. The speed of sound in gas, however, is much slower than in soft tissue, and in bone it is much higher. Gas is also much less dense than soft tissue, and bone is much more dense. Therefore there are large changes in both the density and the speed of sound, so the difference in Z is huge.

SPECULAR AND NON-SPECULAR REFLECTIONS

Interfaces give rise to two types of reflections, specular and non-specular.

Specular reflections occur when the interface is larger than the sound beam. One of their properties is that the angle of the reflection is equal to the angle of incidence. We are all familiar with a common type of specular reflection: a pool ball on a pool table. If we shoot the ball against one of the cushions, it will bounce off at the same angle at which we shoot it (assuming, of course, we are not doing anything fancy like putting a spin on the ball). If we shoot it head on into the cushion, it will come directly back at us; if we shoot it at an angle it will not come back to us.

Figure 1–3 illustrates specular reflections as they pertain to ultrasound.

It is obvious that unless the ultrasound beam strikes a specular reflector nearly head on, the echo will not come back to the transducer but will go angling off into the tissue. The scientific expression for this is that the echo has an "angle dependence." This simply means that the strength of the echo depends not only on the difference in acoustic impedance at the interface but also on the angle at which the beam strikes the interface.

Specular echoes are very common in abdom-

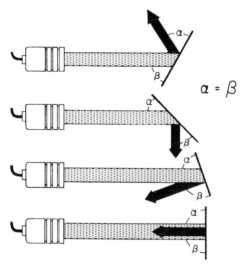

$\alpha = \beta$

Figure 1–3. Specular reflections occur when the reflecting interface is larger than the sound beam. The angle at which the echo is reflected is equal to the angle at which the pulse hit the reflector. The echo will return to the transducer *only if* this is a right angle or very close to it.

inal scanning. The capsules of the liver and kidney, the aorta and major vessels, the gallbladder, and the bile ducts are all examples of specular reflectors.

Specular echoes are something of a problem in gray-scale ultrasound. One of the goals of gray-scale scanning is the preservation of echo amplitude information. Each shade of gray corresponds to a certain range of echo amplitude and might be expected to be the same every time this type of echo is received. But since the amplitude of a specular echo depends not only upon the nature of the interface but on the angle as well, it is clear that the shade of gray will vary widely, depending upon where the transducer is positioned when the echo is received. Thus, the echoes from the capsule of the kidney may be stronger, the same as, or weaker than the echoes from the renal parenchyma, depending upon the beam angle. There is no way to avoid this problem; however, it is not too difficult to live with as long as we recognize that the shade of gray of a specular echo does not have much significance.

Non-specular reflections occur when the interface is smaller than the sound beam. As we shall see, the sound beam from a modern, well-focused transducer is on the order of 3 mm in diameter. Therefore, interfaces smaller than 3 mm will give rise to non-specular reflections. Many small parenchymal tissue echoes fall into this category, such as those arising between cells and small vessels, hepatic cells and fat cells, and renal cells and renal tubules. In contrast to specular echoes, the amplitude of a non-specular echo is not dependent on the beam angle. That this should be so is obvious if we consider that the small non-specular interface is always surrounded by the beam and hence there really is no such thing as an incident angle as far as the interface is concerned. Although not dependent on the angle of incidence, the amplitude of non-specular echoes is usually much less than the amplitude of specular echoes—usually by at least 30 dB—because the interfaces are so much smaller and consequently cannot reflect as much of the beam as the larger specular interfaces.

Gray-scale scanning makes good use of these reflections. Because the differing amplitudes of many echoes are recorded in different shades of gray, it is possible to scan at the high-gain settings required to receive non-specular echoes and still maintain a useful image. Since the echo amplitude is independent of beam angle, the shade of gray (corresponding to the amplitude) of an echo is more nearly constant and more diagnostically useful.

BIOLOGIC EFFECTS OF ULTRASOUND WAVES

High-intensity ultrasound waves can permanently alter the structure of the tissue through which they pass. These effects range from slight warming of the tissue to total necrosis and destruction. The power levels that produce these changes are many orders of magnitude greater than the power levels used for diagnostic B-scanning, however. The power output or intensity of the ultrasound beam is measured in watts per square centimeter (W/cm^2) when biologic effects are being considered. There has been extensive research on the safety of ultrasound in recent years, and no adverse effects have ever been demonstrated at intensities less than 100 milliwatts (mW) per square centimeter (a milliwatt is one thousandth of a watt). The peak intensity, that is, the intensity at the height of the pulse, for present ultrasound B-scanners is less than 100 watts per square centimeter. Since the pulse is actually on about one one thousandth of the time (the remainder of the time the scanner is "listening for the echo"), the temporal average intensity is only a thousandth of the peak intensity or less than 100 mW per square centimeter. Actually the latest generation of gray-scale scanners have temporal average power output of about 20 mW per square centimeter.

The American Institute of Ultrasound in Medicine established a Committee on Biologic Effects to study the problem of possible toxic effects of ultrasound scanning. In August, 1975, this committee issued the following statement, which summarizes the knowledge of the biologic effects of diagnostic level ultrasound:

Statement on Mammalian in Vivo Ultrasonic Biologic Effects

In the low megahertz frequency range there have been (as of this date) no demonstrated significant biologic effects in mammalian tissues exposed to intensities* below 100 mW/cm. Furthermore, for ultrasonic exposure times† less than 500 seconds and greater than one second, such effects have not been demonstrated even at higher intensities, when the product of intensity* and exposure time† is less than 50 joules/cm.

---

*Spatial peak, temporal average as measured in a free field of water.
†Total time; this includes off-time as well as on-time for a repeated-pulse regime.

All of the commercially available ultrasound scanners have power outputs well within this safety range.

PERSPECTIVE

It is time to stop and count heads; we have made it through the worst of the physics and we hope that no one got lost along the way. From now on the discussions will be more practical in orientation, but we will often refer to the physical principles we have just been over. At the risk of beating a dead horse, we want to reiterate that it is impossible to be a good ultrasonographer unless you have some understanding of where the echoes come from and why; only then can the more subtle problems, such as artifacts, be comprehended and dealt with; only then can the ultrasound literature be read with enough understanding to separate the valuable articles from the trash; and only then can scanning techniques be modified and improved.

BIBLIOGRAPHY

Kremkau, F. W.: *Diagnostic Ultrasound: Physical Principles and Exercises.* Grune & Stratton, New York, 1980.
(A very nice, short, understandable physics book; it even has test questions so you can see how you are doing.)

Who's Afraid of a Hundred Milliwatts Per Square Centimeter? American Institute of Ultrasound in Medicine, Washington, D.C., 1979.
(This little pamphlet, written by members of the AIUM bioeffects committee, is an excellent short summary of the biologic effects problem. It is available from the AIUM office.)

Chapter 2

TRANSDUCERS AND RESOLUTION

Strange bedfellows, you say; what do transducers and resolution have in common? Everyone knows that resolution should be discussed in physics chapters, and besides, all you need to know about resolution is that higher frequencies mean better resolution; and this means, of course, that all you need to know about transducers is the higher the frequency the better, right? Yes and no. Although resolution is a "physics" topic, we believe it is far too important to be buried in a physics chapter. And while it is generally true that higher frequencies *can* produce pictures with better resolution, there is a big gap between theory and reality. The claims of ultrasound systems salesmen notwithstanding, there is far more to resolution than frequency; in fact, the frequency number stamped on the side of the transducer is probably the *least* useful indicator of its resolving capability. It is true, however, that the characteristics of the transducer govern the resolution of the system; and that is why we are going to discuss them together. We chose the chapter title to be deliberately provocative. We want to be certain that everybody remembers that *resolution is determined by the design of the transducer and its supporting electronics. The mode of scanning, real-time or static B-scanner, has nothing to do with resolution.*

There is a widespread misconception (often espoused by people who really should know better) that static B-scanners have inherently better resolving capability than real-time scanners. Not true. Indeed, there is considerable difference in the resolution capabilities of different scanners, but this is due to the design and construction of the machines and is not related to whether they are real-time or static. At the time of this writing, from the standpoint of resolution the best two machines commercially available are both real-time units. The worst two are also real-time units. Static B-scanners occupy the middle territory; and while the general trend is toward improved resolution

by all scanners, the gap between the best and the worst seems to be widening. It is important, therefore, that everyone have a good understanding of transducers and how their design and construction affect the resolution of the ultrasound image; without this knowledge it is impossible to make an intelligent decision as to which machine to buy or use for a particular scanning situation. Fortunately the concepts are easy to understand; we will start with the most basic and work our way through to the most sophisticated.

THE PIEZOELECTRIC EFFECT

The term *piezo-* is derived from a Greek word meaning pressure, so *piezoelectric* translates into *pressure-electric*. This refers to a property of certain crystals that causes them to emit electricity when pressed or deformed. Conversely, when electricity is applied to a piezoelectric crystal it changes the shape of the crystal.

This phenomenon has many uses besides ultrasound. One with which many of us are familiar is the phonograph. When amplified record players first became available, a piezoelectric crystal was attached to the needle, and this crystal generated the small electric currents that were then amplified and played over a loudspeaker. (For the most part, crystals have been supplanted by magnetic cartridges in present-day stereo systems)

Figure 2–1 illustrates the piezoelectric effect as it is exemplified in an ultrasound transducer. When a high voltage, between 300 and 700 volts, is applied to opposite faces of the crystal, it expands slightly. If the voltage is turned off the crystal returns to its original size. If the voltage were reapplied, but with opposite polarity (that is, if the positive and negative electrodes were switched), the crystal would shrink slightly. These tiny expansions and contractions

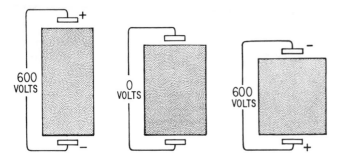

Figure 2-1. When a voltage is applied to it, a piezoelectric crystal either expands or contracts, depending upon the polarity of the voltage. Conversely, if the crystal is physically compressed or stretched, it will generate a voltage in the electrodes.

of the crystal generate the small pressure waves that are transmitted as the ultrasound pulse. When the crystal is placed in contact with the patient's skin, these expansions and contractions cause pressure waves in the tissue and create the ultrasound beam. When an echo returns to the crystal the small pressure waves deform it slightly, causing a tiny voltage to appear in the electrodes. The greater the amplitude of the echo, the more the crystal is deformed and the higher the voltage generated. (This voltage is in the range of 0.01 to 1000 mV [1000 mV = 1 volt], quite small when compared with the large voltage used to initiate the pulse.)

Short quiz: If the echoes received from a typical abdominal scan generate voltages ranging from 0.01 to 1000 mV, what range of echo amplitude does this represent in decibels?

Answer: Recall the definition of the decibel:

$dB = 20 \log \frac{E_2}{E_1}$. A factor of 10 is equivalent to

20 db. To go from 0.01 mV to 1000 mV requires five factors of 10, so this is equivalent to 100 dB. This could also be calculated directly as:

$$20 \log \frac{1000}{0.01} = 20 \times 5 = 100 \text{ dB}.$$

There are several types of crystal that possess piezoelectric properties. Quartz is an example of a naturally occurring piezoelectric crystal, but many synthetic materials also have piezoelectric qualities and have several advantages over quartz. At present virtually all transducers for medical ultrasound purposes are made of lead titanate zirconate, although the exact recipes for various models differ, and many of the details of their construction are industrial secrets.

There is one practical matter to keep in mind when dealing with synthetic crystals: the effect of heat. Synthetic piezoelectric crystals are constructed by crystallizing a ceramic material in the presence of a strong electric field. This "polarizes" the crystal and makes it piezoelectric. If the crystal is reheated in the absence of an electric field it can lose its polarization. For this reason, transducers should never be heat-sterilized.

FREQUENCY

The frequency of a transducer is determined by how many times the crystal expands and contracts per second. There are two ways of controlling this.

The first simply involves cycling the voltage applied to the crystal at whatever frequency is desired. If we wanted a 2.5 MHz transducer, we would cycle the voltage 2.5 million times per second; if we wanted 3.5 MHz, we would cycle at 3.5 MHz. (Although this may sound difficult, it is actually quite simple for the electronics circuit designer.) There are some advantages to controlling frequency this way. To begin, we know exactly what the frequency is. Also, if we wanted to change frequency, we could simply turn a dial and change the excitation rate without having to touch or change the transducer. Some Doppler systems use this type of excitation of the crystal.

There is a major problem with using this method in pulse-echo systems, however, and that is pulse length. As we shall see, the axial resolution of the ultrasound system is limited by the pulse length; to get high resolution we must have a very short pulse, ideally only a single cycle. This is not possible if an oscillating voltage is used to drive the crystal at a fixed frequency. Fortunately, there is a method of controlling crystal frequency while maintaining short pulse lengths; this makes use of the property known as resonance.

Resonance is defined as a reinforcement of sound by sympathetic vibration. This definition probably seems a bit obscure, and it is easiest to understand resonance by considering some everyday examples.

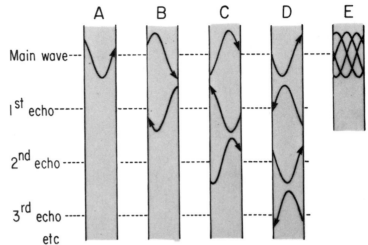

Figure 2–2. When the wavelength is not related to the size of the vibrating object, the effective amplitude may be nearly zero. *A* to *D* show how the main wave and some of the echo waves generated as internal reflections, or resonance, occur. In this diagram we have shown each wave on a separate line for simplicity. Actually, all the waves are superimposed, as in *E*, and tend to cancel each other out.

We are all familiar with musical glasses. After an elegant meal someone lines up all the partially empty wine glasses and starts banging on them with a knife. The glasses "ring" when struck, producing a tone with a definite pitch. Each glass, however, produces a different tone, depending on how much wine it contains—the more wine, the higher the pitch. If the dinner guest is musically inclined, he can often play a tune on the glasses. How is it that identical wine glasses can produce different notes when struck by the same knife? Resonance, of course. When the glass is struck it starts to vibrate, and the vibrations produce pressure waves in the air, which we hear as sound. The pitch of the sound depends on the frequency at which the glass is vibrating. The amount of wine in the glass determines the frequency of the vibrations and hence the pitch of the note.

A xylophone works on exactly the same principle. The wooden bar of the xylophone is struck with a stick and starts to vibrate. The vibrations produce pressure waves in the air, which we hear as sound. The pitch of the sound is deter-mined by the frequency at which the bar vibrates, and this frequency is determined by the size of the bar. Similarly the pitch of a guitar string depends on its length because the length determines the frequency at which the string vibrates.

In an ultrasound transducer the crystal is "shocked" by a single extremely short pulse of electricity (analogous to striking a xylophone bar with a stick or plucking a guitar string). The crystal then vibrates or "resonates" at a frequency determined by its thickness.

Advanced study department: The physical principles behind resonance are beyond the scope of this book. Figures 2–2 and 2–3 are a brief attempt to illustrate how this phenomenon works. If you are still confused, do not lose any sleep over it. From a practical, clinical standpoint all you have to know is that the frequency of a transducer is determined by its thickness because of a physical phenomenon known as resonance. For those who want more we suggest you refer to a general college physics or ultrasound physics text.

Figure 2–3. When the size of the vibrating object is one half a wavelength the effective amplitude of the wave is increased. *A* to *D* show the main wave and some of the echo waves generated by internal reflections, or resonance. In *D*, we have shown each wave on a separate line for simplicity. Actually, all the waves are superimposed, as in *E*. The resulting amplitude is the sum of all the waves and is increased.

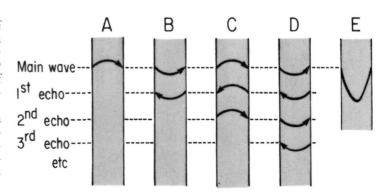

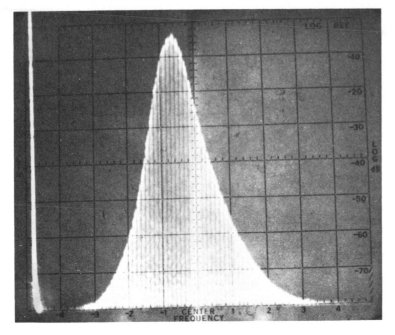

Figure 2–4. The frequency spectrum of a modern transducer can be quite narrow. This is the actual spectrum of a transducer with a nominal "frequency" of 2.25 MHz. The largest portion of the output is between 1.5 and 3.0 MHz. The peak frequency is 2.15 MHz, and each horizontal scale division is equal to 0.5 MHz. (Courtesy of Aerotech Laboratories).

BANDWIDTH

Under ideal circumstances a transducer would emit sound waves at only a single frequency, determined by its crystal thickness. In practice, however, this is not possible. Slight imperfections in the crystal, non-parallel faces, irregularities in the face, coupling of waves into the load and backing material, length of exciting pulse, and many other factors all combine to broaden the frequency of the transducer. (Sometimes these factors are deliberately manipulated so that the transducer will have a large frequency spectrum.) Even though a transducer is designed to operate at a single frequency, it actually emits ultrasound waves of many frequencies on either side of the main frequency. The range of frequencies produced is known as the bandwidth of the transducer. A transducer with a large bandwidth emits many different frequencies. There have been considerable technical advances in transducer construction in recent years, and modern transducers can have quite narrow bandwidths. Figure 2–4 shows an actual spectral analysis of an ultrasound transducer. Most of the frequencies produced are closely grouped about the peak frequency of 2.15 MHz. There is no significant output at frequencies of 1.0 and 3.5 MHz.

Transducers are labeled with the frequency that corresponds to the peak of the bandwidth curve, but this does not tell us very much about the actual output. As Figure 2–5 illustrates, the peak of the curve may have little to do with the effective output, and just because one transducer is labeled with a higher frequency than another does not mean it will actually perform better. In fact, it is the presence of a wide bandwidth that permits transducers labeled "5 MHz" to make pictures of the abdomen. As we shall see in the next section, it is impossible for

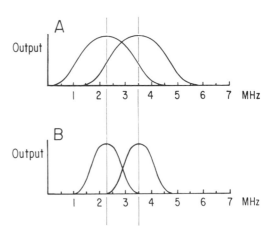

Figure 2–5. If transducers do not have narrow bandwidths, there may be little difference in the pictures they produce.

A. The bandwidths of a 2.5 and 3.5 MHz transducer overlap significantly because they are so wide. There is little difference in the actual sound beam.

B. Because the bandwidths are narrow, these 2.5 and 3.5 MHz transducers have very different outputs.

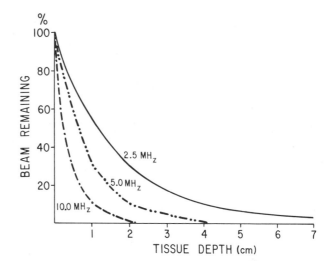

Figure 2–6. Higher frequencies are attenuated much more rapidly than low frequencies. The graph shows the percentage of the beam remaining at various tissue depths for three different frequencies. See text for more details.

a 5 MHz sound beam to penetrate more than 5 or 6 cm of tissue, yet at least one company has been very successful marketing "5 MHz" abdominal scanning systems. Since that machine does make pictures (and pretty good ones, too), it is apparent that the transducer has a very wide bandwidth, and it is the low-frequency components of the beam that are producing much of the image.

BEAM "SOFTENING"

Remember in Chapter 1 when we calculated the attenuation coefficients for various frequencies? We found that attenuation was directly proportional to frequency; that is, as the frequency increased the attenuation increased. Thus a 5.0 MHz beam will be attenuated twice as rapidly as a 2.5 MHz beam. Figure 2–6 is a plot of the attenuation of the ultrasound beam

for three different frequencies: 2.5, 5.0, and 10.0 MHz. Each of the beams starts off at 100 per cent power, and the curves show how much is left for recording an echo from various tissue depths.

There are two things to notice. First, attenuation takes a big toll from all the beams. Even the best, the 2.5 MHz, has been depleted to only 5 per cent at a depth of 6 cm. Second, and most important, the higher frequencies are more severely affected. Only 1 per cent of a 5.0 MHz beam is left for an echo from 4 cm, and a 10.0 MHz beam is effectively gone by 3 cm. This means that as the ultrasound beam passes through tissue its high-frequency components are quickly filtered out and only the low frequencies are able to penetrate to the tissue depths—8 to 10 cm—required in abdominal scanning. Figure 2–7 illustrates the effect on the output of the beam by comparing a bandwidth spectrum at the skin line and at 6

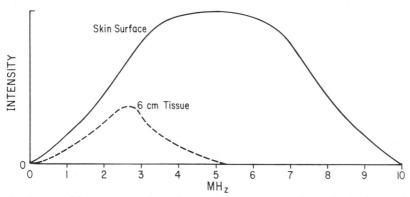

Figure 2–7. As the sound beam passes through tissue its spectrum is changed: The higher frequencies are selectively absorbed and the beam is "softened." The solid line shows a hypothetical 5 MHz transducer beam spectrum at the skin surface. The dashed line shows the spectrum of the same beam at 6 cm tissue depth.

cm of tissue depth. We call this shift to lower frequencies as the beam passes through tissue "beam softening." The word *soft* comes from general physics nomenclature, which terms high frequencies "hard" and low frequencies "soft." (The opposite effect occurs in diagnostic x-ray exams; the lower frequencies are selectively attenuated, and the x-ray beam "hardens" as it goes through tissue.)

Beam softening is a fact of life in the ultrasound world; all ultrasound beams are subject to it regardless of what any machine salesman tells you. If the transducer is making pictures at a depth of 8 or 10 cm it is not doing it with a 10.0, 7.5 or 5.0 MHz sound; this simply is not possible. The "7.5 MHz" stamped on the transducer is either fiction or (more likely) represents the center of a wide bandwidth.

IMPEDANCE MATCHING

Since the first edition of this book there have been tremendous improvements in transducer design and manufacture (which account for much of the improvement in image quality during the last five years). One of the most significant innovations has been the development of impedance matching.

The density difference between the face of a transducer and the soft tissues of the body is very large. This results in a large impedance mismatch, and consequently a large portion of the ultrasound beam is reflected off the skin surface and never makes it into the body. **Impedance matching** refers to any process that lessens or minimizes this initial reflection. Different manufacturers use different methods to accomplish this. In the main they involve coating the transducer face with a polymer (plastic) that is intermediate in density between transducer and tissue. This reduces the size of the impedance "mismatch" between transducer face and skin, and enables a larger percentage of the sound beam to pass into the body. In addition, by varying the thickness of the polymer, the resonant properties of the beam can be improved. There are different proprietary names for impedance matching; the most widely known is "quarter-wavelength technology." Regardless of the name, virtually all the major manufacturers use some method of impedance matching to improve the output of the transducer, and the results have been impressive. The signal-to-noise ratio and the output of present transducers are markedly superior to their predecessors.

AXIAL RESOLUTION

There are two types of ultrasound resolution, axial and lateral. **Axial resolution** refers to the resolution *along the path* of the beam. As the beam travels through tissue it encounters numerous interfaces: How close together can these interfaces be spaced and still be distinguished? The answer is usually expressed in millimeters and is called the axial resolution; the smaller the number the better the resolution.

Comparative terminology department: In evaluating radiologic systems, resolution is usually expressed in terms of line pairs per distance rather than simple distance; in this case the *larger* the number of line pairs, the *greater* the resolution.

Although axial resolution depends on many factors, by far the most important is the pulse length.

Physical principles state that axial resolution can be no better than half the pulse length. Figure 2–8 illustrates why this is so. The pulse length is easy to calculate; it is simply the duration of the pulse times the speed of sound in tissue. The speed of sound is 1540 meters per second, and a typical ultrasound pulse lasts between 1.5 and 2.0 μsec; thus a typical pulse length is about 2 mm. This means that the best possible axial resolution· is on the order of 1 mm for most modern scanners. (Of course, machines do not actually achieve this "best possible" result because of other "weak links" in the system.)

A short pulse length is obtained in two ways. The first involves physically "damping" the crystal by placing absorbent material behind it. Recall how the cymbal player cuts short the crash of the cymbal by grabbing it with his hand; he has "damped" the vibration. Nearly everyone is familiar with the "damper" pedal on a piano (the one on the right). When this pedal is pressed the piano strings are free to vibrate, and notes will be sustained for several seconds. When the pedal is released the strings are "damped" (by bringing a felt pad into contact with them), and the sound is extinguished. The same principle is applied to ultrasound transducers; an acoustically absorbent material is placed in back of the crystal to cut short any ringing and limit the pulse length.

An even more effective means of limiting the pulse is electrical damping, which involves reversing the polarity of the transducer crystal to stop its motion. This is analogous to a pilot reversing the thrust of the jet engines as soon as the plane has touched down on the runway

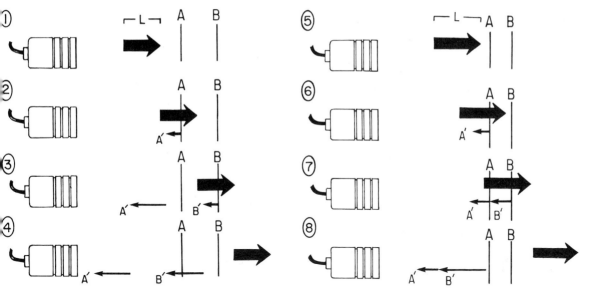

Figure 2–8. Diagrammatic representation of the effect of pulse length on axial resolution. Lines 1 to 4 show the situation in which two interfaces, A and B, are separated by more than half the pulse length, L. The echoes from A and B (A′ and B′) do not overlap, and the transducer sees two separate echoes.

Lines 5 to 8 show the situation when A and B are closer than one half of L. In this case, the echoes A′ and B′ overlap and the transducer sees only a single echo.

to slow it down quickly. Nearly all current machines use some type of electrical damping to limit the pulse length.

How short can the pulse length go? In theory, it could be made infinitely small and resolution infinitely great. As always, there is a Catch-22. If the pulse gets shorter than one wavelength there is no vibration at all and no pulse can be produced. It is not possible, therefore, to decrease the pulse length to less than one wavelength. Here is where frequency comes into the picture. The higher the frequency, the shorter the wavelength; consequently a higher frequency can produce a shorter pulse and provide better axial resolution.

Another limitation of decreasing pulse length is the broadening of the bandwidth; as the pulse gets shorter the bandwidth gets wider and the effects of beam softening become more pronounced. We cannot have our cake and eat it too. Efforts to improve resolution by increasing frequency run into penetration and bandwidth problems. This has led many manufacturers to turn away from the single multipurpose machine and concentrate on designing scanners to serve special purposes. The most familiar example is the special limited-range, high-resolution scanner, generally referred to as a "small parts scanner." These machines concentrate on high frequency and have traded off penetration

for improved resolution in a limited range, usually no more than 3 to 4 cm.

LATERAL RESOLUTION

Lateral resolution refers to resolution perpendicular to the axis of the sound beam. It can also be thought of as side-to-side resolution. As the beam is swept through tissue it encounters many interfaces located side by side at the same depth: How close together can these interfaces be spaced and still be distinguished? Like axial resolution, lateral resolution is expressed in millimeters, and the smaller the number, the better the resolution. Lateral resolution depends on the width of the sound beam, as is illustrated in Figure 2–9. If two interfaces are closer together than the beam width, they will both give rise to an echo at the same time and only a single echo will be received by the transducer.

The expression *beam width* can be very nebulous. Although we use it frequently and probably have a good intuitive notion of what it means, it is not so easy to make a precise definition. The ultrasound beam is similar to a paint sprayer; there is no sharp edge. Although the sprayer will deposit most of the paint in a small circle, there will be some paint sprayed

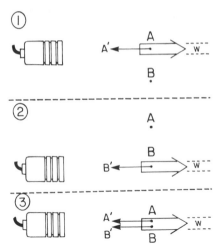

Figure 2–9. Lateral resolution is limited to beam width. If interfaces A and B are separated by more than the beam width, W, then, as the transducer is moved across them, two separate echoes A′ and B′ will be generated (lines 1 and 2). However, if A and B are closer together than the beam width, the echoes A′ and B′ will arrive at the transducer simultaneously and be recorded as a single echo (line 3).

over a wider area. What constitutes the "size" of the paint spray? Is it where 30 per cent of the paint is sprayed? 50 per cent? 90 per cent? Clearly we must pick some arbitrary amount— say 50 per cent—and define the "size" of the spray as that area in which 50 per cent of the paint falls.

A similar arbitrary definition of ultrasound beam width must be selected. Instead of using the amount of sound (which is what we did with the paint) we use the amplitude of the sound beam. Thus we say the beam "ends" when the amplitude decreases by 3 dB, or 6 dB, or 100 dB. The width of the beam will vary depending on which level is chosen, as illustrated in Figure 2–10.

If 3 dB is chosen, the beam will appear to be very narrow, since this represents only a 30 per cent reduction from peak amplitude. This, however, is not a particularly useful definition for our purposes. Since the echoes we are receiving cover a range of 100 dB, a change of only 3 dB is hardly noticeable. A 20 dB beam width is a more useful definition, and 40 dB is even better. The point to keep in mind is that when the beam widths of two transducers are compared, it is important to know how the beam width is being defined. (The same problem occurs in describing the power of stereo equipment; the "watts" of one manufacturer may not be equal to the "watts" of another.)

About face department: Now that we have warned you about putting too much stock in any descriptions of beam widths we will proceed to examine various types of transducer designs and illustrate the resulting sound beams with diagrams, as though they were precisely defined. These pictures are meant only to describe the shape of the various beams to allow you to compare the effective focus of the different transducer types.

NON-FOCUSED TRANSDUCERS

If the face of the transducer is flat and placed directly in contact with the patient (with no intervening lens system), the transducer is said to be non-focused. The earliest ultrasound scanners all used non-focused transducers, and much has been written describing the resulting beam pattern and width. With the development of focused transducers in the mid-1970's the non-focused model fell into well-deserved obsolescence. Consequently, non-focused transducers are no longer used in modern abdominal and obstetrical scanners.

Non-focused transducers suffered from a wide beam width and severe nonuniformity of the beam in the near field (the area close to the transducer face). Wide beam meant poor lateral resolution—2 or 3 cm was average—and nonuniformity meant that echo amplitude was not

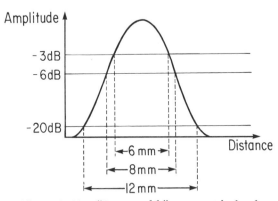

Figure 2–10. "Beam width" varies with the decibel level used to define it. In this example we are examining a single beam profile. The amplitude of the beam is plotted on the vertical axis versus distance on the horizontal axis. If we define the beam "width" as 3 dB (this means the beam "ends" when it has decreased 3 dB in amplitude), the width is 6 mm. If we call 6 dB the end of the beam (this corresponds to a 50 per cent loss of amplitude), the width is 8 mm. At 20 dB (a reduction of 90 per cent) the width is 12 mm.

reproducible and the gray scale had little meaning. The fixed-focus transducer improved this situation.

FIXED-FOCUS TRANSDUCERS

As is the case with visible light, ultrasound waves can be focused by using lenses. The actual physics of this process is quite complicated and not really important for their clinical use; we need only keep a few basic principles in mind.

To begin, focusing greatly improves the characteristics of the beam by decreasing its width and making it more uniform. Since the lens is round, the beam is focused in all directions. This means that the thickness of the beam and consequently the thickness of the ultrasound "slice" is reduced. A modern fixed-focus transducer can have a beam width as small as 3 to 5 mm.

One-upsmanship department: The sophistication of modern CT scanners permits resolution of a millimeter or less *in the scan plane,* yet the thickness of the slice is usually 7 mm or more. In these situations ultrasound wins the resolution race.

The larger the diameter of the transducer face, the more precisely it can be focused. Most modern static B-scanners use a 19 mm transducer that can be more effectively focused than the 13 mm transducer used in older machines. If the transducer were made larger, the focusing could be made even better. In addition, as the transducer face is made larger it can collect more sound and detect lower-amplitude echoes. Unfortunately it is not practical to use very-large-diameter transducers, since it is difficult to keep a larger, rigid area in contact with the patient's skin. (Some manufacturers are getting around this problem by scanning through a water path; this allows them to use transducers as large as 8 cm in diameter.)

Increasing the frequency of a transducer also improves its focusing characteristics. But we have already seen that attenuation makes the use of frequencies much greater than 3.5 MHz impractical for abdominal and obstetrical scanning.

The degree of focusing can be controlled by varying the construction of the lens. Figure 2–11 shows the beam profile from two transducers, one focused in the near field and the other in the midrange. Which is better? It is hard to give a definite answer. A tightly focused

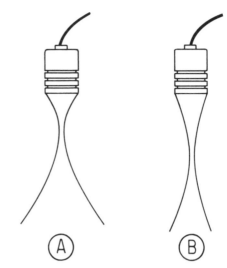

Figure 2–11. The focusing of a beam is not uniform throughout the range.
A. The transducer is focused in the near field and the beam widens considerably in the far field.
B. The transducer is focused in the midrange and has better focus than A in the far field.

beam produces the best resolution (as little as 2 or 3 mm) in its **focal zone** (the imprecisely defined but intuitively obvious area of maximum focus). The beam, however, does not perform well outside the focal zone. As the beam is focused farther from the transducer face, the focal zone becomes longer. The short-focus transducer will produce better pictures in the near field, but its resolution in the mid and far fields will be inferior to that of the transducer that is focused deeper. No transducer can be focused well in the very near field—the area within 2 cm of its face.

The **focal length** (the distance of the focal zone from the transducer face) is controlled by the way the lens is constructed. Thus it is possible to have a set of tightly focused transducers of different focal lengths; one for the near field, another for the middle zone, and a third for the far field. By selecting the transducer with a focal zone in the area of interest we can make pictures with the best resolution. This requires us to own several transducers. More importantly, we must be willing to change them according to the needs of each examination. Nevertheless, this is the way to get the best results from a static B-scanner, and after all, if we are going to the trouble of doing the examination at all we should always do the best job even if it involves the inconvenience of juggling transducers.

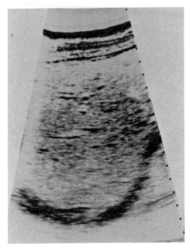

Figure 2–12. The beam is "hotter" in the focal zone than in the near and far fields. The apparent increased intensity of echoes in the middle of the liver occurs because the sound beam is more concentrated and intense in the focal zone.

Focusing a transducer produces an artifact in the image with which we all need to be familiar. As the beam is made smaller it is also concentrated and its intensity increases. For this reason echoes from the focal zone appear louder than those from the near and far fields. Figure 2–12 illustrates this phenomenon. Some of this can be corrected by pre-image signal processing in the scanner (discussed in Chapter 3), but we have yet to see a machine that compensates perfectly for this artifact of focusing.

The modern fixed-focus transducer is a sophisticated piece of equipment that produces pictures of far higher quality than its predecessor of three or four years ago. Still it has some limitations; it cannot be focused in the very near field and, unless a water path is used, makes very poor images in this region. Also, because it is "fixed-focus," the focal length cannot be varied, and we must change transducers to look at different tissue depths. Finally, focusing produces the intensity artifact discussed in the preceding paragraph. For these reasons there has been considerable interest in another type of transducer—the phased-array or "electronically-focused" transducer.

LINEAR PHASED-ARRAY TRANSDUCERS

The concept of the phased-array transducer is not new—it was first introduced in the early 1970's as a method of producing a real-time image—but it was not until the latter part of

the decade that engineers began using this principle to improve the focusing and resolution of the transducer. The earliest phased-array transducers had very poor resolution. Despite this, many were sold as real-time units and achieved some popularity, especially among obstetricians. Unfortunately the bad resolution was blamed on the real-time feature instead of on the fact that these scanners were using primitive unfocused transducers. The current linear phased-array transducer is a different beast from the early models and is capable of producing a highly focused beam with resolution rivaling that of the fixed-focus transducers.

The physical principles involved in the phased array are mind-boggling, sufficient to cause seizures in even the most diligent student. We will greatly oversimplify their operation so that we can get a general idea of how they work.

Rather than being a single round crystal, these transducers are composed of thin rectangular chips lined up side by side as shown in Figure 2–13. Each chip has its own circuitry and functions as an independent mini-transducer. The final product resembles a large pack of chewing gum in which the individual sticks are analogous to individual transducer chips. The total number of chips in the transducer varies from 11 to 128, depending upon the manufacturer; the larger units use the extra chips to create a real-time image, as we shall see in Chapter 3.

Figure 2–14 illustrates how a group of chips can be used to produce a focused beam. (We will show only 5 chips for simplicity; in actual practice most transducers use about 11 chips.) The two outside members of the group are fired first (Figure 2–14A); a fraction of a second later

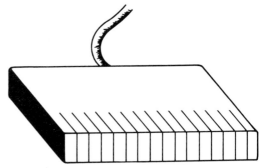

Figure 2–13. The linear phased-array transducer is constructed from several small individual crystals lined up side by side like sticks of gum in a package. Each element has its own circuits and can be fired independently or in combination with other crystals.

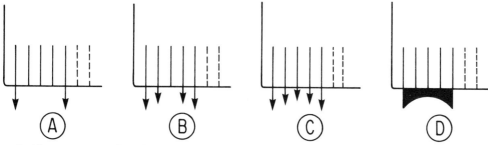

Figure 2–14. By varying the time at which individual crystal chips are fired, an "electronic lens" can be created. See text for details.

the two adjacent ones are fired (Figure 2–14*B*), followed in another fraction of a second by the center chip (Figure 2–14*C*). This slight delay causes the center of the sound beam to lag behind the outer edges as shown in Figure 2–14*C* and produces the same effect as if the beam were passed through a lens (Figure 2–14*D*). In fact, it is probably easiest to think of this whole process as the creation of an "electronic lens" for focusing the beam. The focal zone of the "electronic lens" can be altered by changing the timing at which the individual chips are fired (Figure 2–15). Thus the transducer can be focused in the near, middle, or far field by electronic manipulations in the scanner itself; there is no need to change transducers to change the focal zone.

The most common type of linear phased-array unit is the familiar "bar," which is very popular as a low-priced real-time scanner. (As we mentioned before, the earliest versions of

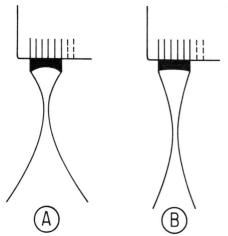

Figure 2–15. The shape of the "electronic lens" can be varied by changing the timing of the firing of the elements.
A. The "lens" is focused in the near field.
B. The best focus is in the far field.

this instrument did not use phased focusing and made pictures of poor quality; now many manufacturers offer the more sophisticated focused version.) A second type of linear phased-array transducer has a smaller number of chips and is physically about the same size as a conventional fixed-focus one. It also produces a real-time scan, but the image is sector-shaped rather than the rectangle produced by the "bar." The resolution of these units has, so far, been inferior to that of the longer "bar"-type scanner.

Linear phased-array transducers are not without their limitations. The "electronic lens" can only be created along the line of the chips, which means that precise focusing can only be accomplished in the plane of the scan; the scan slice is often quite thick. The most advanced units partially compensate for this by using a fixed-focus lens perpendicular to the plane of the scan; still, the resolution perpendicular to the scan plane is not as good as with the conventional fixed-focus transducer.

Linear arrays also are subject to **side lobes**. Side lobe formation is a complex phenomenon that is (very loosely) analogous to the formation of a rainbow. We are all aware that light can be "bent" by passing it through a transparent material such as water or glass. Different wavelengths are bent by different amounts; when the sun shines through a rain cloud and its light is bent, each wavelength (color) is bent a different amount and the colors are separated. In addition, if the sunlight is strong enough the process may occur more than once, and two or even three rainbows may be produced. The second and third rainbows are "side lobes" of the original rainbow. Any transducer with multiple elements is subject to a similar process. The individual elements, or chips, function as a diffraction grating that can bend the sound wave just as water in the rain cloud bends sunlight. This results in a slight separation of the individual wavelengths or frequencies (which is not significant for clinical purposes) and the production of side lobes (which is significant). Just as a second or third rainbow increases the overall width of the rainbow, the formation of side lobes increases the width of the ultrasound beam and decreases the lateral resolution. The details of this process are light years beyond the scope of this book but are covered in modest detail in some ultrasound physics texts. All we need remember is that side lobes are bad news; they decrease resolution and can produce some unusual artifacts as well. The side lobe problem can be lessened, but not eliminated, by using sophisticated electronic filters in the processor circuits of the scanner. Side lobes are especially bad in the small "sector" type of phased-array transducer; so bad, in fact, that this transducer is not really suitable for quality abdominal scanning (although it is adequate for echocardiography in which the resolution and gray-scale requirements are more modest).

ANNULAR PHASED-ARRAY TRANSDUCERS

As we have seen, both the fixed-focus and the linear phased-array transducers have some shortcomings. The annular array transducer is designed to utilize the strengths of both while minimizing their limitations.

In this transducer the individual elements are thin concentrically arrayed rings much like the rings in an onion or a tree trunk. In operation the timing of the rings is manipulated to create an "electronic lens" just as in the linear array; but because the transducer is round, the "lens" focuses the beam in all directions, not just in the plane of the scan. Theoretically this produces not only good resolution within the scan plane but an extremely thin plane as well. The thickness of the slice can be as little as 2 mm. It is also claimed that the annular design reduces the side lobes that haunt the linear arrays.

One currently available annular array transducer is large, 7.5 cm in diameter. Consequently it cannot be placed conveniently in contact with the patient but must be used through a water path.

Socratic method department: Why the large-diameter transducer? Large transducers are more sensitive and can be more effectively focused. This holds for arrays as well as fixed-focus transducers.

This transducer is "dynamically focused"; that is, the maximum focus (about 2 mm) can be adjusted electronically from near to far field by the sonographer. It can also be focused continuously so that the focal zone automatically follows the sound pulse and the transducer is always focused at the depth from which the echo is being received.

SPECIAL-PURPOSE TRANSDUCERS

Tranducers are available in a bewildering variety of sizes, shapes, and frequencies. In addition to those for regular scanning, there are several special-purpose models. These include tiny ones that can be attached to needles or probes, rotating models for insertion into bodily orifices, small-face models, special high-resolution limited-range transducers, and various grooved and channeled types for guided biopsy. The only two of particular interest to the abdominal and pelvic ultrasonographer are the high-resolution limited-range and the biopsy transducers.

High-resolution limited-range transducers are available from several companies and are generally called "small parts" scanners, although it is not clear what constitutes a "small part" (the thyroid? the testicle? the carotid artery? the breast?). It is more precise to consider them as very-high-resolution scanners with a limited range of penetration, usually no more than 3 or 4 cm. The resolution of these machines is impressive—as little as 0.5 mm. This is accomplished by using very high frequencies (8 to 10 MHz) in combination with special electronics to shorten the pulse length. It is the high frequency that limits beam penetration to no more than 5 cm. You will recall that no transducer can be focused in the area close to its face. Therefore these "small parts" transducers are not used in contact with the skin but scan through a water path. This permits the zone of maximum focus to fall in the first 3 cm of tissue (it also reduces artifacts, as we shall see later). All these machines are real-time.

It is obvious that this is a complicated business and the high-resolution "small parts" scanner is far more than just a high-frequency transducer plugged into a general abdominal scanner; it is a completely separate scanning unit.

There is no such thing as a free lunch department: Do not be misled by some manufacturers' claims of an add-on, inexpensive "small parts" transducer. Many companies offer a high-frequency transducer for their scanners, but in general you will not get 0.5 mm resolution from these units. For optimum performance you must have the special pulse length circuitry and the water path scanning head to get into the very-high-resolution ball game, and unfortunately, at present the price is not cheap.

Biopsy transducers are essentially the same as standard transducers with the addition of a central channel in the axis of the sound beam through which a biopsy needle can be passed. They are available in both fixed-focus and linear phased-array models and produce nearly as good pictures as their standard counterparts.

TRANSDUCERS FOR GENERAL SCANNING

In the first edition of this book we felt that it was necessary to have several transducers in a general abdominal and pelvic ultrasound practice. Improvements in transducer design and focusing have obviated the need for a large number of separate transducers, and most laboratories should now need only two. The key factor is the focal zone; you must be able to produce high-resolution pictures at any tissue depth. If you are working with transducers whose focal zone cannot be changed (and this means all static B-scanners and most real-time

units) you will need a general purpose model focused at around 4 to 8 cm and a second focused in the near field (2 to 6 cm). The near-field transducer can be higher-frequency than the general one, since the sound beam does not have to penetrate so much tissue. As we have seen, the "official" frequency of a transducer does not always give an accurate description of its output. Although 3.5 MHz is the highest frequency that can penetrate to the tissue depths encountered in abdominal scanning, 5 MHz can be used for tissue depths up to 6 cm. If you want to do very-high-resolution imaging of superficial structures, you will have to lay out the considerable extra money for one of the "small parts" scanners.

Finally, you may want to add a biopsy transducer. We no longer use ours, despite the fact that we do many biopsies (we have developed a simple form of triangulation that is as accurate in most cases and a lot less trouble in all cases).

We have spent a long time discussing the different types of transducers. Nevertheless, we want to stress that the transducer is only one part of the overall imaging process. Picture quality depends not only on the transducer but also on the quality of the ultrasound scanner, the type of electronics and image display, the nature of the patient, and most importantly, on the skill of the person performing the scan. All the transducers in the world cannot compensate for poor scanning technique.

BIBLIOGRAPHY

Hefner, L. V., Parks, J. A., and Goldstein, A.: Transducer beam pattern test object. *Journal of Clinical Ultrasound* 8:5 (1980).
(This paper has excellent illustrations and a discussion of beam focusing patterns and the effect of side lobes.)

Kremkau, F. W. *Diagnostic Ultrasound: Physical Principles and Exercises.* Grune & Stratton, New York, 1980.
(A very nice, short, understandable physics book; it even has test questions so you can see how you are doing.)

Chapter 3

SCANNERS

When we wrote this chapter for the first edition five years ago, life was simpler. There were only a half dozen scanners on the market and they were all pretty much peas in a pod, real-time was still a novelty with limited use in abdominal scanning, and digital image storage and processing were on the drawing board. Times have certainly changed. It is almost impossible to find an analog scanner, real-time is displacing static scanning as the preferred technique, and there are as many different kinds of scanners as there are companies in the market. We will not go into detail on the individual workings of every machine available, but we do want to explore the basics of scanner operation that are common to them all and point out the major differences between the varying approaches to real-time scanning. We will take a look inside a "typical" scanner and see what happens to the sound pulse during its journey from the patient's body to the ultrasonologist's mind. Figure 3–1 is a block diagram of the important components in a scanner and can serve as our road map for the trip. There are three major divisions of a scanner: the image production system, the storage system, and the display system.

IMAGE PRODUCTION SYSTEM

Pulses

Our first step in generating an image is to send out the ultrasound pulse. Remember that the pulse is generated by "striking" the crystal with a very brief electric shock—half a microsecond or less—which sets the transducer crystal vibrating at its resonant frequency. In order to get good axial resolution, however, we must keep the pulse length short; therefore, most scanners employ some form of "reverse shock" or electrical damping to snuff out the vibrations quickly and limit the pulse duration. If our machine uses a simple fixed-focus transducer then this single electric shock and damping are all that is required. If we are using the more sophisticated array transducers, however we will also need a complex electronic network to alter the timing of the shocks to individual transducer elements to create a focused beam.

How often can we repeat the pulse? Here we are limited by the speed of sound—there must be enough time for the pulse to travel to the interface and return before starting a second pulse; otherwise our echoes will pile up on top of each other. Now, at 1540 meters per second the pulse will travel 1.54 mm per microsecond. It follows, then, that if we want to be able to receive an echo from a distance of 20 cm we must allow 260 μsec for the sound pulse to make the journey to the interface and back (total distance traveled is $2 \times 20 = 40$ cm $= 400$ mm; 400 mm $\div$ 1.54 mm/μsec $= 260$ μsec). The maximum pulse rate we can use will be about 3800 pulses per second. This is certainly rapid enough for manual scanning in which the rate of image acquisition is a snail's pace (most manual scanners pulse at a rate of 1000 per second); but as we will see, it limits our picture size in real-time.

Preamplifiers

Now we have our pulses going out, and the echoes are returning to the transducer. When an echo strikes the transducer face it deforms it slightly, and this generates a tiny electric voltage. Just as the echoes are very small when compared with the size of the outgoing pulse, the electric voltages they generate in the transducer are also tiny, ranging from 0.05 mV to 1000 mV (lest you get carried away, remember that 1000 mV is only 1 real volt—that little AAA battery in your electronic baseball game generates 1.5 volts). In order to do anything with these small voltages we are going to need some amplifiers.

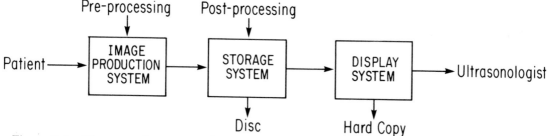

Figure 3–1. There are three major divisions in an ultrasound scanner. The image production system collects and analyzes data from the patient and sends it to the storage system. The information may be processed further before going to the display system where it is viewed by the ultrasonologist.

The first job is to get the signals back to the scanner from the transducer; they are too small to make the trip by themselves, so we will help them out by using a preamplifier. The preamplifier can be located either in the scanner itself or out in the transducer head; regardless of location, its role is to boost the strength of the tiny voltages from the crystal and send them to the main scanner for processing and analysis. This is not an easy task, because the range of echoes is very large, and it is important that their strength not be distorted by uneven amplification. A very sophisticated conglomeration of electronic hardware is required to produce a linear amplification response across such a long range.

Comparative acoustics department: Many of us are familiar with stereo amplifiers and the considerable hoopla and hype with which their responses to low and high frequencies are promoted. Our range of echo voltages is from 0.05 to 1000 mV (90 dB), which is comparable to the 10 to 25,000 Hz range of sound frequency in the highest-quality stereo systems.

Time Compensated Gain (TCG) Amplifier

If there were no attenuation of the ultrasound beam in tissue, a simple preamplifier would be adequate for our scanner. As we saw in Chapter 1, however, the beam is attenuated by approximately 1 dB per centimeter per megahertz. This means that the echo from an interface will become weaker, the farther the interface is located from the transducer.

Figure 3–2 illustrates a hypothetical scanning situation. A 2 MHz ultrasound beam is scanning a homogeneous tissue that has the same attenuation coefficient as human soft tissue (1 dB/

cm/MHz). There are only three interfaces in our hypothetical tissue; one is located 3 cm from the transducer, the second is 6 cm from the transducer, and the third is located at 9 cm. All three of these interfaces have the same acoustic impedance dance mismatch; that is, they would all give rise to the same amplitude echo if they were located the same distance from the transducer. Since the interfaces are at

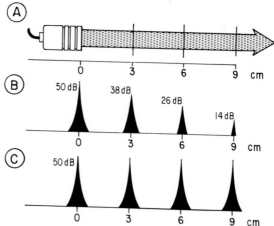

Figure 3–2. Echoes from deep interfaces are attenuated to a greater extent than echoes from near interfaces.

A. A 2 MHz ultrasound beam is directed through three interfaces located 3, 6, and 9 cm from the transducer. Each of these interfaces is the same and would give rise to a 50 dB echo if there were no attenuation of the beam.

B. Because of attenuation, the echoes become progressively weaker. This line shows the amplitude of the echoes as they are received by the transducer.

C. To compensate for the loss of echo amplitude, time compensated gain (TCG) is used. TCG amplifies the deeper echoes more than the near echoes and restores each echo to its original 50 dB.

different depths, however, they will not give rise to echoes of equal amplitude because the echo from the deeper interfaces will be attenuated to a greater extent than the echo from the closest interface. Now suppose that, in the absence of any attenuation, this interface would yield an echo of 50 dB. What amplitude echo will be received from the interfaces at 3, 6, and 9 cm? Since we are using a 2 MHz beam, the attenuation will be: 2 MHz × 1 dB/cm/MHz = 2 dB/cm. The echo from the interface at 3 cm will have traveled 6 cm overall (3 going and 3 returning) and will have been attenuated: 6 cm × 2 dB/cm = 12 dB. Similarly, the echoes from the interfaces at 6 and 9 cm will have traveled 12 and 18 cm and will have been attenuated 24 and 36 dB respectively. Thus the echoes received from these three interfaces would be (50 − 12) = 38, (50 − 24) = 26, and (50 − 36) = 14 dB.

Notice that although attenuation is dependent on frequency and distance, it does not depend on the basic amplitude of the echo. Weak and strong echoes will be attenuated the same amount. In the example of Figure 3–3 the attenuation is the same whether the original echo had an amplitude of 50 dB or 36 dB. (If the original echo indeed had an amplitude of 36 dB, what would be the amplitude of the received echo from the interface at 9 cm? Could we detect this echo? Read on for the answer.)

Since attenuation depends only on distance and frequency, it is possible for us to compensate for this loss of amplitude by using differential amplification. All we need to do is to amplify echoes more if they come from a greater distance. Consider again the echoes in Figure 3–2, line B. Now we know that each of these echoes is supposed to have an amplitude of 50 dB. Yet the received echoes had amplitudes of 38, 26, and 14 dB. This means we must amplify the echo at 3 cm by 12 dB, the one at 6 cm by 24 dB, and the one from 9 cm by 36 dB. If we do that, then all three echoes will emerge from the amplifier with an amplitude of 50 dB (Figure 3–2, line C), and we will have corrected for attenuation. (How would this work if the original echo were 36 dB? Pretty well, for the 3 and 6 cm interfaces; the echoes from these would be restored to their original 36 dB. The echo from 9 cm, however, was attenuated to 0 dB and hence was never detected by the transducer. Thus there is no way we can amplify it, and this echo would remain undetectable.)

This concept of correcting for attenuation by using differential amplifications is known as **time compensated gain**, or TCG. (In the world of ultrasound *gain* is synonymous with *amplification* and is a lot easier to write and say.) The *time* refers to the fact that the amplifier automatically increases the gain as a function of time. But time is the same as distance in ultrasound. (Remember way back when we met the man who measured canyons by shouting across them? He repainted his watch face so that it read in distance instead of time. Therefore, TCG really stands for *distance compensated gain*.

We are all ready to add TCG to our amplifier, but how should we set it up? What rate of compensation should we use? If we knew that only a 2.25 MHz transducer was going to be used, then we could set it for the average attenuation, which is: 2.25 MHz × 1 dB/cm/MHz = 2.25 dB/cm. This would not work so well with a 3.5 MHz or a 5.0 MHz transducer, however. It also might not work well with a 2.25 MHz transducer if the attenuation were much different from average. For instance, a cirrhotic liver has a very high attenuation rate and would require more compensation than average. A pregnant uterus has less than average attenuation and would need yet another setting. The obvious solution is to allow the ultrasonographer to select the TCG that is appropriate for the scanning situation. (We will discuss the operation of this control in Chapter 5.)

The TCG amplifier limits the overall sensitivity of the ultrasound scanner. At a scanning frequency of 2.25 MHz an interface only 10 cm deep (not at all uncommon in abdominal work) would need 45 dB of TCG to avoid distortion. Some amplifiers simply aren't capable of producing this, and hence they cannot record weaker echoes from these distances. When a 5 MHz transducer is used the TCG requirements are immense; 50 dB at 5 cm. Since TCG is added to the baseline amplification, which must be capable of 90dB to record the range of normal echoes, ideally the total range of the amplifiers should be on the order of 140 to 150 dB. Continued improvements are being made in them, but amplifiers represent a limiting factor in the sensitivity of ultrasound scanners.

We should also notice that the TCG requirements are independent of transducer performance. That is, even if the transducer were perfect—a tightly focused beam with no loss of intensity due to dispersion—TCG would be necessary, since attenuation is caused by the tissue itself. In practice, transducers are not perfect and the beam tends to be weaker in the far field, adding an even greater burden on the TCG amplifier.

In addition to handling a wide range of incoming echoes, the TCG amplifier must compress the echoes into a smaller output range. The subsequent signal processing electronics and the storage system are not capable of dealing with 90 dB, and so the output of the amplifier is compressed down to 30 to 40 dB. This is usually done logarithmically, which means that the larger the echo, the greater the amount of compression. Thus an echo of 90 dB might be chopped down to 30 dB, (a reduction of 60 dB), while an echo of 10 dB is reduced to 4 dB (a loss of only 6 dB). Some manufacturers use other methods of compression, such as thresholds or sinusoidal transforms; the details are not important as long as you understand that the raw echo signals undergo considerable modification and that they are not all changed the same. On some scanners the operator can make adjustments in the way the echo compression is carried out; this is a form of preprocessing, which we will discuss in a moment.

Before leaving the topic of amplifiers and gain we should say a word about "overall" or "system" gain. This simply refers to the general level of gain that is applied uniformly to all echoes, regardless of strength. This controls the overall intensity of the echoes in the picture and is analogous to the volume control on a stereo system. (We will discuss this further in Chapter 5.) In most modern scanners the system gain control operates the preamplifier, but some scanners incorporate an additional amplifier after the TCG to handle this function.

Echo Quantification

Our echoes have now been correctly amplified and compressed, but they are still in the form of an electric signal. The next step is to convert the electric voltage into a number that measures the amplitude of the echo. Actually the problem is a little more complicated than this; the scanner must first separate all the echoes from each other and decide exactly where they begin and end. The echoes are strung together like a long freight train, and the scanner must uncouple the train so that it can count the individual cars. Several different electronic processes are available to accomplish this, the details of which need not concern us. Names attached to these manipulations are *rectification*, *demodulation*, *detection*, *differentiation*, *integration*, *peak analysis*, *peak picking*, and others. Whatever the term, the end result is the important thing; using a variety of processes that we shall lump under the general heading of "echo quantification," the scanner identifies and measures the amplitude of the echoes.

The term *preprocessing* is frequently bruited about these days. Translated, this simply means any modifications that are made in the echo information in the *pre*-image process. The most obvious example of preprocessing is the TCG amplifier and its controls; we electronically change the appearance of the final image by selectively amplifying distant echoes to compensate for attenuation. The compressing of echoes from 90 dB down to 30 dB is another example of preprocessing. Other parts of the quantification process can also be varied to create a change in the appearance of the final image. Some preprocessing is hard-wired into the scanner, and some is under the control of the ultrasonographer. TCG, for instance, is always under the control of the machine operator. Similarly, many manufacturers allow the ultrasonographer to select from several different compression amplification curves. Some machines permit minor modifications in the quantification process. Others try to compensate for the change in beam intensity that occurs with focusing. With the exception of TCG, most of the preprocessing options make little difference in the final image. If your particular machine offers them it is fun to play around to see the effect on the final image, but we doubt if anyone does this after the initial excitement wears off. It is probably best to choose whatever settings give an image pleasing to your eye and leave them there.

Once the echoes have been processed and quantified they are ready to be sent to the image storage system. Almost all machines sold today (except for the most inexpensive, which don't have any storage system) use a digital memory for storage. A digital memory can only accept whole numbers as input data; and, therefore, our quantitative echo amplitude information must be rounded off to whole numbers before it is sent to storage. This is done with a neat little "black box" device known as an A/D converter.

One-upsmanship department: This is pronounced "A to D converter" and stands for analog to digital. A/D converters are a notoriously weak link in the electronic chain, and if you want to appear knowledgeable to your service man, you can always whip off a casual, "It may be in the A/D converter."

Of course, we have only the echo amplitude information at this point; we still need to determine where in space the echo originated (the storage system needs this information so that it may properly position the echo in the image.) This requires some type of position monitor.

Position Monitor

There are three different modes of display used in diagnostic ultrasound: A, B, and M. B-mode is used in clinical abdominal and obstetrical ultrasonography. A-mode and M-mode have been the basis of echocardiography, but even here, B-mode is rapidly becoming the preferred method.

A-mode (the *A* stands for amplitude) is the simplest form of display. Figure 3–3 illustrates this type of presentation. We are displaying only two parameters of the echoes: their distance from the transducer and their amplitude.

The distance is shown along a horizontal line, while the amplitude is depicted as vertical deflections from this line. The big problem with A-mode is that the ultrasonographer must know where the sound beam is pointed, and this is very difficult except in the most simple of scanning situations. The image just looks like an ever-changing range of mountains, and it is usually impossible to glean much anatomic data from the A-mode display. (There are a few diehards who still occasionally use this presentation just as there are still some people who bake their own bread. Unlike home-baked bread, however, A-mode is a vastly inferior product.)

M-mode is basically A-mode with a minor variation. A-mode measures the position and amplitude of the echoes, while M-mode records the position and the motion of the echo (the *M* stands for motion). To make M-mode we first start with the A-mode display. Each spike on the display is then replaced with a single dot. The brightness of the dot is made proportional to the amplitude of the echo. Now if all the echo-producing interfaces are stationary, the dots will remain stationary; but if one of the interfaces is moving (such as a heart valve or the wall of the aorta), the dot corresponding to that interface will also move. If the interface moves back and forth toward the transducer, the dot will also move back and forth toward the transducer.

To record this motion we can do one of two

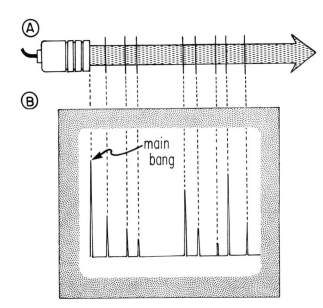

Figure 3–3. A-mode displays the echoes as a function of distance from the transducer.

A. An ultrasound beam passing through several interfaces.

B. The A-mode display of the echoes as they would appear on an oscilloscope. The oscilloscope trace starts with the "main bang," which corresponds to the transducer face. Each echo is displayed as a spike; the height of the spike is proportional to the amplitude of the echo. The distance from the main bang to the spike is proportional to the distance from the transducer to the interface.

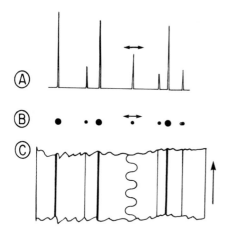

Figure 3–4. M-mode records the motion of echoes.

A. An A-mode display of echoes.

B. To obtain M-mode, the spikes are replaced with dots; the brightness of the dot is proportional to the height of the spike and the amplitude of the echo.

C. If an interface is moving the dot will also move and the motion of the dot can be recorded by running a light-sensitive paper in front of the display. Dots that are stationary produce straight lines while dots that move produce wiggly lines.

things: either we can slowly move the line of dots across the face of the oscilloscope from bottom to top or we can slowly run a photographic film or light-sensitive paper in front of the line of dots. Either method will produce the same image—a series of lines. Each line corresponds to an echo interface. Interfaces that are stationary will produce straight lines, while moving interfaces will produce wiggly lines. The wiggly line represents the motion of the echo with time. Figure 3–4 illustrates M-mode.

B-mode is the mainstay of abdominal and pelvic ultrasonography. The *B* stands for brightness. This is not a particularly good description, and if we were naming things over we would call it P-mode to signify "picture." Figure 3–5 illustrates how this works.

First we start with the A-mode display and replace the spikes with dots, just as for M-mode. The brightness of the dot is made proportional to the amplitude of the echo; the louder the echo, the brighter the dot. Now instead of orienting the dots from left to right on the oscilloscope screen, we will have the line of dots oriented in the same direction that the transducer is pointing. When the transducer is moved, the line of dots corresponding to the echoes will move in the same direction. The

display system will keep a record of all the dots so that, as the transducer is scanned across the patient, all the echoes that are produced from the various interfaces will be displayed and recorded in the position from which they were produced. This concept is perhaps a little difficult to understand when put into words, but is actually quite easy to grasp visually. Reference to Figure 3–5 will probably be helpful.

B-mode yields a two-dimensional picture of the area covered by the transducer. The amplitude information is maintained in the brightness of the dots. The picture actually represents a "slice" of the patient; the thickness of the slice will be equal to the width of the ultrasound beam. It is this ability to produce a two-dimensional image that makes B-mode scanning so useful to the ultrasonographer.

The first gray-scale scanners were static B-scanners in which the transducer was mounted

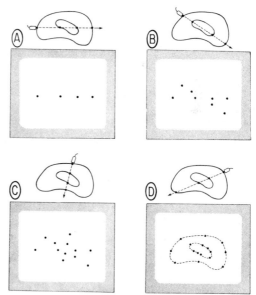

Figure 3–5. B-mode generates a "picture" of the area being scanned. The echo spikes in the A-mode presentation are replaced with dots; the brightness of the dot is proportional to the amplitude of the echo. Instead of orienting the dots on a horizontal axis, as is done in A-mode and M-mode, the dots are oriented in the same position and direction as the transducer. As the transducer is scanned across the patient, the dots will build up an image of the interfaces within the patient.

A to D. The top portion of each figure shows the orientation of the transducer on the patient, while the bottom portion of the figure shows the resulting image on the oscilloscope.

at the end of a hinged arm system. The ultrasonographer moved the transducer within the scan plane and created the image by hand. Electronic devices at the pivot points in the arms kept track of the orientation of the transducer as a pair of coordinates, which were sent, along with the echo amplitude information, to the storage and image processing system.

Real-time scanners are B-scanners in which the transducer moving process has been automated and speeded up. The transducer is still confined to a single scan plane, and its position is still monitored by electronic devices and sent to the storage system along with the amplitude data, but its motion is automated. This means that many frames can be scanned every second and that a continuous or "real-time" image can be produced. The ultrasonographer controls the orientation of the scan plane by hand while the machine moves the transducer within the plane.

Confusing terminology department: Many people confuse B-mode and real-time, feeling that B-mode refers to a static scanner and that real-time scanners somehow do not produce a B-mode picture. Any scanner that produces a two-dimensional image is a B-mode scanner, or "B-scanner." All real-time scanners are B-scanners. The correct distinction is between **static** (any machine in which the transducer must be moved in the scanning plane by hand) and **real-time** (machines in which the sound beam is automatically and rapidly moved in the scan plane.)

A bewildering variety of real-time scanners is available today; however, they are all variations of two basic designs. In the first type an image is produced by moving the transducer *mechanically*. In the second the sound beam itself is moved *electronically* while the transducer remains stationary. This is not as confusing as it sounds. Let us look a little more closely at these instruments.

Mechanical Real Time

The simplest way of creating a real-time image is by mounting the transducer on a pivot and oscillating it back and forth with a motor as shown in Figure 3–6 (the so-called "electric toothbrush" method). These scanners produce a pie-shaped image (known in mathematical circles as a sector), and, therefore, are most commonly called "sector scanners." There are several variations on this simple theme.

For example, some manufacturers set the transducer back from the skin surface by using a water path; this means the tip of the sector is

no longer in the image and the shape of the scan becomes trapezoidal.

Amateur engineering department: What is the advantage of moving the transducer away from the skin surface? We learned one reason in Chapter 2: No transducer can be focused close to its face, so the immediate near field is an ultrasonic no-man's-land. By backing the transducer off from the skin, this zone of poor focus can be taken out of the patient and the image. Also, larger transducers can be used, and we remember that the larger the transducer, the better the focusing potential. Finally, the extra distance increases the focal length of the transducer and its depth of field. We shall learn yet another reason in Chapter 4.

In some machines the transducer is fixed and the sound beam is deflected off an acoustic mirror. The mirror is then oscillated to move the sound beam and produce the real-time image (Figure 3–7).

Another variation involves mounting the transducer on a wheel that is rotated, as shown in Figure 3–8. Several versions of this type of scanner are available; most use two or more transducers, sometimes with different frequencies or with Doppler capability. Some are contact scanners, while others set the wheel off from the skin with a short fluid path. One machine even has three wheels, each containing several transducers, rotating simultaneously side by side to create a larger image.

Regardless of the specifics of the motion, all mechanical scanners have two traits in common:

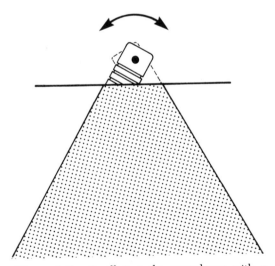

Figure 3–6. Oscillating the transducer with a motor produces a real-time image shaped like a sector. This method is known as the "electric toothbrush" approach to real-time scanning.

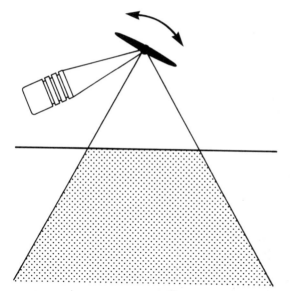

Figure 3–7. A variation of the "electric toothbrush" method involves a fixed transducer: The beam is moved by reflecting it off an oscillating mirror.

They use annular (round) transducers (and therefore can easily focus the beam in a complete 360-degree circle), and they have a fixed focus.

The exception that proves the rule department: One company offers a mechanical real-time scanner that uses an annular array transducer the focus of which can be changed, but more about this later.

Electronic Real Time

Nothing moves in the electronic real-time scanner; rather the ultrasound beam is swept through the patient by changing the firing sequence of the elements in the transducer. The most popular electronic real-time scanners are linear arrays. These are the bar-shaped transducers, which are actually composed of between 64 and 128 tiny individual transducer chips lined up side by side.

Recall that, in Chapter 2, we saw that by altering the timing of activation of the individual chips it was possible to create an ultrasound beam that behaved as if it has passed through a lens. (If you do not recall, go back and look at Figure 2–14 again.) It is easy to see how, by applying the same principle, we can move the beam. Look at the transducer array in Figure 3–9. Suppose we fire only five chips at a time to create the ultrasound beam. We will start by activating the five chips at the left end of the bar (numbers 1 to 5 in Figure 3–9) and produce a single ultrasound pulse. To make the next pulse we will not use the same chips; instead we shift everything one chip to the right and fire numbers 2 to 6. For the third pulse we once again shift to the right and utilize chips numbers 3 to 7. Each succeeding pulse originates one more step to the right until the end of the bar is reached, at which time we return to the left end of the transducer and start over. The effect is the same as if we had mechanically

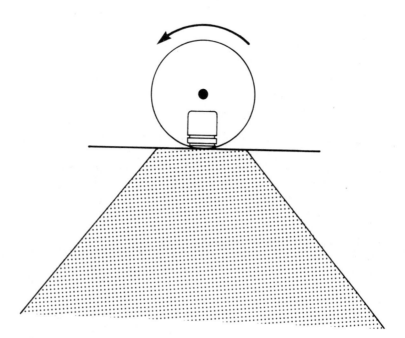

Figure 3–8. Rolling wheels are popular as real-time scanners. One or more transducers are mounted on a wheel, which is turned by a motor. The resulting image is sector shaped.

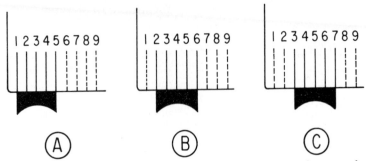

Figure 3–9. The ultrasound beam can be swept down a linear array to produce a real-time image.
A. Elements 1 through 5 are fired, producing a beam centered on chip 3.
B. The second pulse, centered on chip 4, is made by activating elements 2 through 6.
C. The third pulse is centered on chip 5. Each subsequent pulse is moved one element farther down the array.

moved the beam along a straight line, yet the transducer itself has not moved. Since we can create well over 1000 pulses a second, it is possible to make several complete sweeps per second and have a real-time image.

The linear array transducer produces a rectangular picture rather than the sector produced by the mechanical scanners. The rectangle gives a bigger picture area, particularly in the near field, but it also requires a large area of contact between the transducer and the patient. This is not such a problem in obstetrical scanning but can sometimes pose difficulties higher in the abdomen where the ribs can prevent contact of the rigid transducer face with the patient's skin. We also remember that the linear array transducer can be focused well only in the plane of the scan and is subject to side lobe formation, which creates artifacts in the image. Finally the lateral resolution of these scanners is limited by the thickness of the chips because that is the smallest increment the beam can be moved; some type of smoothing or averaging must be used to fill in the spaces or the picture can be rather coarse.

Linear array scanners do have some pluses, however. They are relatively simple instruments with no moving parts to synchronize, stabilize, or wear out (a truly "solid-state" device). This means they are cheaper to manufacture and require little service; consequently they are usually priced much lower than the mechanical scanners. (The simplest of these scanners does not even use a storage system or signal processing but sends the data straight to the display). They can be made compact and portable for use in more than one location, as for example, an office and a hospital. These instruments have become very popular for obstetrics, in which the large field of view is helpful and sophisticated storage and signal processing are not usually necessary.

It is possible to make a sector scanner using electronic beam sweeping with a linear array transducer. In this case the transducer is small and contains fewer chips. All the chips are fired for each pulse, but the timing is staggered from one side to the other, and this results in a beam that is swept across the field. The resolution of these instruments is poor compared with that of the other machines we have been discussing, and the complicated electronics makes them expensive. (Phased-array sector scanners were developed for echocardiography, in which the rib cage makes it imperative to have a small transducer and in which ultrafine resolution and gray scale are not so critical.)

Image Size

All real-time scanners have one undesirable feature in common: The size of the image is small. So small, in fact, that the ultrasonographer often gets the frustrating feeling that he is looking into the patient through a keyhole. If the companies are so clever that they can make dynamically focused array transducers, digital storage, big- time amplifiers, post-image processing, and who knows what other fancy stuff, why not give us a bigger picture? It's against the law—the laws of ultrasound physics, that is.

The problem is the speed of sound. Remember that ultrasound travels at 1540 meters per second in the body. While this seems to be very fast (an ultrasound pulse could run the Boston Marathon in 27 seconds), it is actually a snail's pace in the world of real time. Let's analyze the situation. Suppose we want to get echoes from a depth of 20 cm. We know that we must wait for one ultrasound pulse to go out that 20 cm and return to the transducer before we can send out the second pulse. Since 1540 meters per second is the same as 1.54 mm per microsecond (divide everything by 10^6) it will take 260 μsec for each pulse to make this trip (total distance is 40 cm or 400 mm; divide this by 1.54). At 260 μsec per trip the fastest we can pulse is 3846 lines per second (1 second divided by 260 μsec). Now if we want to have 30 frames per second—the common flicker-free frame rate used in television and motion pictures—each frame can only contain 128 lines (3846 divided by 30). Therefore we only have 128 lines of information to spread over the entire picture. If we spread the lines out too much the lateral resolution will go to pot (since we can't resolve anything smaller than the line spacing) so to preserve the ability to resolve 1 mm echoes we will need at least 10 lines per centimeter and the picture cannot be wider than 12.8 cm (128 divided by 10).

We have been considering an ideal case. In actual practice it is not possible to pulse this rapidly, since the transducer requires time for activation and damping, and the pulses must be spaced far enough apart so that the electronic circuitry has time to analyze, quantitate, process, store, and display them. If some type of water or fluid delay is used, this will increase the distance the pulse has to travel and will further decrease the maximum pulse rate. These factors all combine to limit the rapidity with which lines of information can be collected and, consequently, how many lines are available for each frame. We can spend the lines however we choose, but it always involves a compromise. If we make the image size larger we will either have to spread the lines farther apart (decreasing the resolution) or we will have to settle for fewer frames per second (and a flickering image).

Each manufacturer has approached the problem differently, but most have made resolution their top priority, which means that the size of the image has been kept relatively small. (One company allows the ultrasonographer to vary the picture size and resolution to suit the situation; another has an automatic circuit to shrink or expand the picture size, depending on the depth of penetration desired; a third allows the ultrasonographer to decrease the frame rate so that the resolution can be improved.) The small image size is certainly a problem with real-time scanners. In actual use, however, the other advantages of real-time scanning outweigh this limitation. In Chapter 5 we will see how proper scanning technique minimizes the problem of the small field of view.

Time to regroup department: We are finally ready to resume our journey through the scanner. It may have been a little confusing here in the image production system because there are so many different types of scanners on the market. They all reach the same point, however; they have ready to go to the storage system a signal that consists of a number, representing the amplitude of the echo, and a pair of coordinates orienting that echo within the scan plane. From here on the machines are pretty much the same.

STORAGE SYSTEM

Digital Information

It is unlikely that there is anybody left who is not familiar with the term *digital*—it seems to have replaced *space-age* as THE word of the eighties. We all know it has something to do with computers, but we need to go into a little more detail if we are to have a clear understanding of how it affects our final ultrasound image.

Contary to popular belief, computers are not smart; in fact, they are pretty dumb. What they can do well is add and subtract zeros and ones, compare two numbers to see which is larger, and remember great quantities of numbers. But they can do this very quickly, and that is what makes them useful. Although limited to elementary thought processes, they can perform millions of operations a second and, through a process of trial and error, find correct answers much faster than the more sophisticated human brain. Because they do all their thinking with numbers they are called digital devices, and their input and output must be in the form of whole numbers.

Most of the rest of the world operates with continuous or "analog" information. Ultrasound pulses, electric signals, oscilloscope and television phosphors, film emulsions, and the human eye are all analog systems. (We are all familiar with the difference between analog and digital watches; this is an excellent way of conceiving the subtle differences between analog and digital information.)

For most uses analog information is superior to digital information; it permits wide ranges of data to be appreciated in a continuous spectrum. For example, in digital mode we might have 64 different gray shades, but in analog the number is theoretically limitless. Then why have digital memories replaced the analog scan converter in ultrasound scanners? Two reasons: First, analog scan converters are generally very delicate and unstable, require frequent service, and have short life expectancies. Second, and more important, analog signals cannot be modified and stored rapidly or well. Once in digital form, ultrasound information is available for computer processing and storage at high speed, and this offers vast potential for improving our perception and use of the data. Virtually all modern ultrasound scanners use a digital storage and processing system.

Digital Memory

We have our ultrasound information in the form of three numbers: an amplitude (or strength) measurement and two coordinates (or position) in the scan plane. The digital memory is like a large checkerboard on which the scanning plane is superimposed. Figure 3–10 shows a very small memory with only eight rows and eight columns, a checkerboard with 64 squares. Each square in the checkerboard can be identified by its row and column number as shown in Figure 3–10A. As echoes are received in the memory they are assigned to whichever box in the checkerboard most closely approximates their location in the scan plane. Figure 3–10B shows how the echoes from a round cyst would be assigned to the memory. It is obvious that our small memory is not very useful, since the cyst no longer looks round. We do not have enough boxes in the memory to portray the cyst adequately—our matrix is too small. (The term *matrix* refers to the number of rows and columns in the memory. Figure 3–10 shows an 8 × 8 matrix. Each individual box in the matrix is called a *pixel*.) If we had more rows and columns, a larger matrix, we would be able to store the echoes from the cyst more precisely in space and preserve its round shape. Most ultrasound scanners use a 256 × 256 or a 512 × 512 matrix, which enables them to store the image with very little loss of resolution.

Once the location of each echo has been determined, its amplitude is stored in the appropriate pixel in the matrix. Figure 3–10C shows our cyst in final form with each pixel containing a number corresponding to the amplitude of the echo. (Notice that the back wall of the cyst has higher amplitude echoes than the sides or front wall.) The range of amplitude numbers that can be stored is referred to as the "depth" of the memory. A memory that is "four deep" can store 16 numbers.

Computer theory department: How many numbers can a "six-deep memory" store? A "seven-deep memory"? Each layer, or depth, of the memory represents a factor of 2, and so the amount that can be stored in a memory that is "n deep" is given by 2 to the nth power or 2^n. Thus a "four-deep" memory can store $2^4 = 16$ numbers. A "six-deep" memory will store $2^6 = 64$ numbers, while a "seven-deep" memory can hold $2^7 = 128$ numbers.

The earliest digital memories were "four deep" (16 shades of gray), but many manufacturers are now using six- or seven-deep memories (64 or 128 shades of gray).

The larger the memory in terms of matrix size and depth, the more closely it will be able to approximate the analog data and the better will be the resolution and dynamic range (a.k.a. gray scale). In search of the ultimate resolution we could go on expanding the memory size, but we would quickly come to a point at which the memory matrix would have better resolution than the ultrasound beam and there would be no further improvement with increasing size. Similarly, there is not much point in having a very large dynamic range when the human eye can perceive only about 16 shades of gray. With current image production systems a 512 × 512 matrix and 64 shades of gray are more than adequate.

Once the image is stored in the memory, all manner of computer manipulations or post-image processing can be performed. This includes such things as smoothing, edge enhancement, expansion, linear or area histogram analysis, output curve manipulation, linear measurements ("electronic calipers"), area calculation, and the like. Most of these are performed as part of the display process and will be discussed in a moment. At present the clinical value of post-image processing has not been determined, but experience with similar manipulations in CT scanning and nuclear medicine suggest that it may prove very helpful in improving diagnoses.

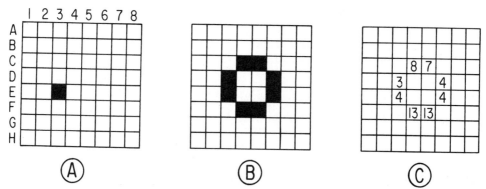

Figure 3–10. The digital memory stores information in a matrix that looks like a checkerboard.

A. A small 8 × 8 matrix with 8 columns (1 to 8) and 8 rows (A to H). An echo has been stored in the matrix at location 3,E.

B. The echoes from a cyst are stored in the matrix; because the matrix is small, the shape of the cyst is somewhat distorted.

C. The amplitudes of the echoes from a cyst have been stored in the memory. Notice that the back wall of the cyst produces louder echoes than does the front wall.

It is a simple matter to transfer digital information for long-term storage. Recently "floppy discs" have emerged as the most convenient medium for storing this data. "Floppy discs" are about the size of a 45 rpm record and can be easily popped in and out of a disc recorder. They are cheap and easy to store. When one wants to recall the images, all that is required is to insert the disc into the scanner or a separate disc player.

IMAGE DISPLAY SYSTEM

We now have our image produced and stored in the memory, but it doesn't do us much good until displayed in some form. There are two devices for doing this: an oscilloscope and a video (TV) monitor.

Oscilloscope Display

An oscilloscope is a cathode ray tube (CRT). A cathode ray tube consists of a gun that shoots a tiny beam of electrons at a phosphor target. When the electron beam strikes the target it causes the phosphor to glow and produces a small dot of light. The brightness of this dot is proportional to the intensity of the electron beam; if the beam is intense the spot will be brighter than if the beam is weak. We can, therefore, feed the amplitude information to the electron beam, and a loud echo will produce an intense electron beam and a bright dot on the phosphor screen. The intensity of the dot

can be varied only over a limited range of about 25 dB in the highest-quality scopes and 20 dB or less in the average oscilloscope.

The electron beam is steered about the target by either electric plates or electromagnets. The position information can be fed to the steering mechanism, and this will assure that the electron beam is properly aimed so that the echoes appear in the correct location. This aiming mechanism is quite precise in an oscilloscope, and very little distortion is introduced into the picture.

There are good and bad points to oscilloscope displays. In their simplest form they are cheap, and some of the inexpensive linear array scanners utilize them for this reason. (These scanners do not even use a storage system; they simply send the signal directly from the image production system to the oscilloscope.) Oscilloscopes have very good spatial resolution and can give better display resolution with less distortion than can video systems. In the highest-quality scopes the dot brightness is very precisely controlled, and this gives a very good gray-scale rendering. On the negative side, cheap oscilloscopes do a poor job of both spatial and gray-scale resolution, and since there is no video signal, it is not possible to make real-time videotape recordings of the display.

Video (TV) Display

A video monitor is similar in many ways to an oscilloscope. There is an electron gun that shoots a tiny electron beam toward a phosphor target. When the beam hits the target it produces a small dot of light, and the brightness of the dot is controlled by the intensity of the beam; however, the beam is not steered in the same manner as in an oscilloscope.

The electron beam in a video monitor starts at the upper left corner and sweeps horizontally across the screen from left to right until it reaches the far side. It then drops down slightly, returns to the left, and makes another horizontal sweep just under the first. This process is repeated until the beam reaches the bottom of the screen; it then returns to the upper left corner and starts all over again. This process is analogous to the way we read the pages of a book: We sweep our eyes across the top line of print, then return and read the second line, and continue until we finish the entire page; then we start again at the top of the next page.

This scanning of the electron beam across the screen is standardized and internally controlled. Although there are several different video formats, all ultrasound scanners use the standard American TV format (the same as commercial television). In this format the beam scans 525 horizontal lines and repeats this process 30 times per second. (Actually the beam scans every other line every sixtieth of a second; this reduces the flicker in the image.)

The spatial resolution of even the best-quality video monitor is not as good as that of an oscilloscope, and there is distortion of the display near the edges (this makes it important to perform all measurements in the center of the picture). Unless an expensive monitor is used, the dynamic range (gray scale) is usually less than 20 dB. Finally, the contrast and brightness of the display are inherently unstable and tend to drift unless special stabilizing circuits are included.

Balanced against these limitations are some very useful features. The brightness and contrast controls allow the ultrasonographer to adjust the picture to best suit the scanning situation and his eye. The video format is easily coupled to video recorders and slave monitors. Many accessories are made for video format. The most frequently used is the familiar alphanumeric display, which allows the ultrasonographer to type the patient's identifying data and other information directly on the image. Because of these convenience features, nearly all ultrasound scanners use the video format for displaying the image.

Thought you caught us up department: Both the oscilloscope and the video monitor are analog devices, and you have been wondering how they handle the digital signal from the storage system, right? Perfectly straightforward. We simply add a digital-to-analog, or D/A, converter between the storage and display system. This is just the opposite of an A/D converter; it changes the digital information from the memory into analog form for the video system.

Post-image Processing

Although post-image processing actually modifies the image while it is in the storage system, we do not see the effects until the image is displayed, and so we have chosen to discuss these options in this section. Post-image processing refers to data manipulations that are performed *after* the image is stored, as opposed to pre-image processing (such as TCG), which is utilized *before* the picture goes to storage.

A simple type of post-image processing is measurement. Electronic calipers are probably familiar to everyone; the ultrasonographer places two dots on the image and the processor calculates the distance between them. Variations include calculation of a circumference or area and the listing of echo amplitudes in a given part of the image (dubbed "histogram analysis" by the manufacturers).

Another common type of post-image processing involves the assigning of a gray-scale map to the amplitude data. Recall that we have stored the amplitude data as a number in the memory; we need to decide how the various

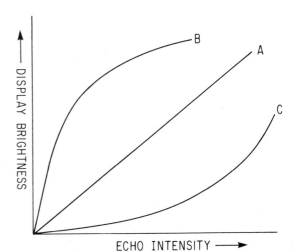

Figure 3–11. A gray-scale map shows how display brightness is related to echo amplitude. Curve A is linear. Curve B accentuates the low-level echoes and produces a contrasty image. Curve C accentuates the high-intensity echoes and produces a "soft" image.

shades of gray are to be assigned to each of these numbers (in computer jargon this is known as constructing a gray-scale map). Figure 3–11 shows three possible ways we could do this. The echo amplitude is plotted on the horizontal axis and the gray-scale brightness on the vertical axis. Curve A is linear and is the simplest: For each unit of increase in amplitude we add a unit of increase in brightness. Unfortunately, the amplitudes of the echoes from abdominal organs are not distributed linearly, and so a linear gray-scale map does not usually produce a very pleasing picture. Curve B is nonlinear, and most of the gray scale has been assigned to the lowest-amplitude echoes. Since abdominal organs produce low-amplitude echoes, this map will create a very contrasty image. Curve C is also nonlinear and has distributed most of the gray scale over the high-amplitude echoes. This curve will cause the organ parenchyma to appear very "flat" or "soft" with little contrast.

There is a limitless number of maps that could be constructed, and they would each give a different appearance to the final picture. Most scanners offer the ultrasonographer three or four from which to choose. Some machines have controls that permit the curve to be continuously varied by changing the slope and origin. One machine allows the operator to set eight different points on the curve, and then the scanner uses these to finish the map.

The effect of changing gray-scale maps is to alter the contrast of the parenchymal echoes in the final picture and to control their brightness. In theory this should enable us to identify subtle variations in tissue texture that might not be appreciated if only a single map or curve were used.

Hard Copy

Hard copy is a term that is applied to any form of picture storage. The most popular type of hard copy for ultrasound images is 8 by 10 inch sheet film (x-ray film). This film has good latitude and contrast; is easy to process, store, and display; and is relatively inexpensive. It is important that the film be exposed to a high-quality image. Many commercial cameras use cheap video monitors, and therefore the quality of the hard copy is often much poorer than the live image on the screen at the time of scanning. This is a serious problem that has been neglected by most manufacturers in the past; they make sophisticated image production and stor-

age systems, and then drop the ball on the one-yard line by not offering a high-quality camera for photographing the end result. Many ultrasonographers are also culpable in this regard. They spend considerable effort producing an elegant image, yet do not take the time to calibrate and adjust the hard copy camera properly. The result is that the beautiful image on the live monitor is very disappointing when seen in hard copy.

Polaroid film has just about passed into extinction as a hard copy medium. The problem is not so much the quality (when properly calibrated, Polaroid film can produce splendid images) but rather the lack of uniformity, the cost, and the inconvenience of mounting and storing the individual pictures.

Floppy discs have already been discussed as a hard copy medium. They are not as convenient as sheet film, since they must be played back through the scanner instead of flipped up on a viewbox. They have the advantage, however, of preserving the digital information, which means that additional post-image processing can be performed after the patient has left.

Videotape is also becoming popular as hard copy, particularly with real-time scanners. As we shall discuss in more detail in Chapter 5, videotape has some uses as hard copy, but we do not feel it should be the primary form of recording or storing examinations; it is too time-consuming to view and too difficult to interpret after the fact.

TGIF department: Finally we've made it through all this physics-y stuff and we are ready to move on to clinical matters. You may not have enjoyed it, but we hope that you will have learned enough about how the ultrasound image is formed so that you can intelligently select and use a modern scanner.

WHICH SCANNER?

There is an old Wall Street joke about the man who goes to a stockbroker saying he wants to make an investment but knows nothing about the market. "Trust me," says the broker, "I know all about stocks; I'll make you rich." A year later the man's stocks are in terrible shape and he has big losses. "Trust me," says the broker, "there are some hot new issues coming out." Again the market declines and the man loses money. "I know what I'm doing," says the broker, "be patient." After a third disastrous year the man asks, "Look, these stocks don't seem to be going so well; should I maybe be investing in bonds?" "Ridiculous!" says the broker, "what do I know about bonds?"

This may not have much to do with ultrasound, but it's a good story with an important point: Do not trust anybody but yourself to decide what type of scanner is best for your practice. We have only four pieces of advice.

1. "Test drive" any machine you consider by scanning yourself. Under no circumstances should you acquire a machine on the basis of only a salesman's pictures or videotapes. The only way to make meaningful comparisons between machines is to see how well they do on a constant, known entity—your abdomen.

2. Technical obsolescence is with us in the foreseeable future; whatever you buy today will almost certainly not be state-of-the-art in two years. This does not mean you should deny yourself the value of a modern scanner, however. After all, even the worst machine on the market today is better than the top of the line in 1978. If you wait for the technical advances to plateau, you may never have a scanner.

3. If possible, observe the use of a scanner on as wide a spectrum of patients as possible. Almost any scanner can make a good picture on those little models the manufacturers are so fond of using for demonstrations. You are interested in how well it can display the entire depth of the right lobe of the liver of a large man.

4. Do not buy a static scanner; these machines are obsolete.

BIBLIOGRAPHY

Winsberg, F.: Real-time scanners: A review. *Medical Ultrasound* 5:99 (1979.)
(An excellent review of the various real-time machines on the market.)

Rose, J. L., and Goldberg, B. B.: *Basic Physics in Diagnostic Ultrasound.* Wiley Medical, New York, 1979.
(Another fairly short, readable physics text for those who want to dig deeper into scanner operation.)

Chapter 4

ARTIFACTS

Before discussing actual scanning procedures we need to examine the problem of artifact production in some detail because it is hard to overestimate the importance of artifacts in day-to-day scanning. Indeed, much of the average ultrasound image is artifact, and in some scanning situations (such as the lower abdomen or pelvis) there is almost nothing but artifact. Five years ago there was very little general awareness of common ultrasound artifacts, particularly those arising from reverberations. In fact, at the 1976 World Congress of Ultrasound in San Francisco there were papers presented in which artifacts were discussed as if they were real echoes. (One particularly memorable presentation discussed a new ultrasonic sign for cancer of the pancreas—but unfortunately the "echoes" the author was describing were all artifact.) Today there is a much higher level of sophistication about ultrasound, and it is unlikely that such obvious mistakes will happen again. Artifacts are still with us, however, and will appear on every scan you perform; it is, therefore, absolutely essential that you have a thorough understanding of what they are, where they come from, what they look like and—most important—how to avoid misinterpreting them as real anatomy.

Exaggerated rhetoric department: Nonsense, you say. If so much of the picture were artifact, ultrasound would have been out of business long ago. Not necessarily. Consider abdominal x-rays. Scattered radiation is, in effect, an artifact on an x-ray film, and an abdominal x-ray frequently contains as much as 50 per cent scattered radiation; the familiar tomogram of the kidneys contains an even greater percentage. The fact that so much of the image is artifactual radiation does not diminish the value of the film for the radiologist because he has learned to recognize the appearance of scatter and to ignore it, concentrating instead on the real parts of the image. Of course he takes steps to reduce scatter as much as possible with grids, high kilovoltage, collimation, and the like. Similarly, in ultrasound, the presence of artifacts need not ruin an image as long as we recognize them for what they are and take steps to avoid them as much as possible.

The most generally accepted scientific definition of an artifact is "something caused by the technique of observation rather than an actual occurrence." This is somewhat obscure, and we prefer to define an artifact in a more general and understandable sense. For our purposes an **artifact** is any part of an ultrasound image that is not a true presentation of the underlying anatomy. There are four types of artifacts that are commonly encountered in abdominal ultrasound: shadows, reverberations, beam focusing effects, and electronic noise.

SHADOWS

Acoustic "shadows" are the major source of "negative" artifacts in the ultrasound image; that is, shadowing causes a decrease in strength, or even complete absence of signals in areas where there are echo-producing interfaces. The term is well chosen because the process is analogous to the shadowing that occurs with light. We have all made shadow figures with our hands in front of a light at some time or other; our hands interrupt the light beam and produce a negative image—a dark pattern—on the wall. Similarly the sound beam can be interrupted by highly reflecting interfaces. When this happens the pulse is unable to reach deeper interfaces, and they cannot produce any echoes to be recorded in the picture. It is not that the interfaces are not there; they are just hidden in the shadow cast by the loud reflector.

By this time you should have no trouble figuring out what type of interface can give rise to acoustic shadowing. In order to cast a shadow, the interface must reflect a large percentage of the sound beam, and this will require a marked mismatch of acoustic impedance (or density)—the kind that occurs with gas and soft

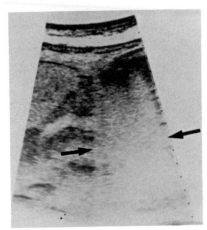

Figure 4–1. Strong interfaces such as air (gas) or bone reflect all of the beam and cast a "shadow" that hides the underlying tissue. In this longitudinal scan the midportion of the aorta and inferior mesenteric vein cannot be seen because they lie in the "shadow" *(arrows)* cast by the air in the overlying bowel.

tissue, or with soft tissue and some much denser material (such as bone, calcium, metal, rubber, plastic). We have already seen how gas causes nearly total reflection of the beam and that it is impossible to "see" through it. Figure 4–1 shows a large shadow cast by air in the bowel that is hiding a portion of the aorta.

Figure 4–2 shows examples of shadowing from soft tissue–dense material interfaces. Although this phenomenon is most commonly seen with calcium (in either bone or soft tissue), metallic surgical clips, rubber catheters or drain tubes, and plastic or metal intrauterine devices (IUD's) will also produce shadows. Even very dense fibrous tissue can give rise to acoustic shadows, particularly if the beam is well focused.

The problem with shadows is that they hide the underlying anatomy from our view. The large shadow cast by air in the stomach usually obscures the tail of the pancreas. Shadows from small bowel air hide the pelvic organs, and the bowel must be pushed out of the way by a full urinary bladder if we are to scan the uterus and ovaries. Shadows from ribs can make it hard to see the upper portion of the liver and spleen. Air in the duodenum frequently shadows the end of the common bile duct.

A more insidious effect of shadowing is the creation of false boundaries and "pseudomasses" as illustrated in Figure 4–3.

Shadows have some redeeming features, however. They tell us that a highly reflective interface is present and we are dealing with either gas or dense material. The vast majority of gallstones cast an acoustic shadow, and this is an important diagnostic criterion in evaluating the gallbladder. Similarly, IUD's will cast shadows, which helps to distinguish them from

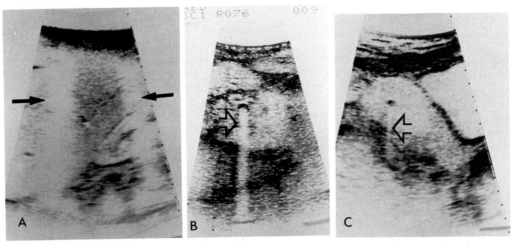

Figure 4–2. Shadows usually arise from either air or very dense material such as bone, calcium, metal, or plastic.

A. The shadows arise from ribs.

B. A calcified renal stone *(arrow)* is casting a shadow.

C. A copper IUD is responsible for the shadow.

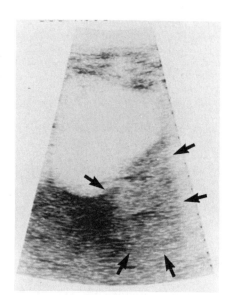

Figure 4–3. Shadows can be mistaken for masses by the unwary. The "mass" outlined by the arrows is not real; it is a pseudomass whose lateral "edge" is created by the shadow from bowel gas.

prominent endometrial echoes. The presence of shadowing in a liver metastasis means it contains calcium and makes the colon the likely primary site.

Refraction

In Chapter 1 we discussed refraction briefly. We called it a slight "bending" of the sound beam as it crosses an interface. Normally the change of direction is so small that it is not recognizable. When the beam traverses a loud echo interface or a series of medium echo interfaces in rapid sequence, it can be displaced enough to produce a "negative" artifact. When the beam is deflected from its true path, the effect is the same as shadowing; there is no sound left to produce an echo from the underlying interfaces. The only place we normally encounter refraction is the side wall of a fluid-filled structure such as the gallbladder or a cyst; small acoustic "shadows" are commonly present beneath their edges as shown in Figure 4–4.

Limited warranty department: The exact mechanisms that produce shadowing from refraction have not been conclusively demonstrated. Some ultrasound physicists believe that refraction is too small

to be apparent in clinical examinations and the "shadows" beneath the gallbladder wall are real, that is, caused by the reflections in the wall itself. Others believe that refraction is a major contributor to all shadows and that reflection of the sound is a relatively minor component. And, of course, there are many who stake out the middle ground. Choose whichever explanation you like; just do not be misled by the shadows when they appear in your scans.

Enhancement

Acoustic enhancement is exactly the opposite of shadowing. If the ultrasound beam passes through tissue with no interfaces (a fluid-filled structure) it is not depleted by echo production and emerges from the tissue with more intensity than would be expected. Thus it will produce louder echoes from the interfaces it subsequently encounters. The resulting increased echo production from underlying tissues is known as acoustic enhancement because the echoes are all "enhanced" by the unattenuated beam. Although enhancement produces "positive artifacts," that is, artifacts that present as increases in echodensity, it rarely causes confusion in diagnosis. In fact, many ultrasonographers use it as a diagnostic criterion of fluid, as we shall discuss in more detail in Chapter 11. Figure 4–5 illustrates acoustic enhancement.

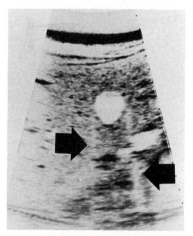

Figure 4–4. Refraction, or bending, of the sound beam can produce the appearance of shadows beneath the side walls of fluid-filled structures.

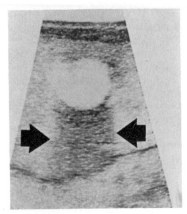

Figure 4–5. Acoustic enhancement is the opposite of shadowing. The sound beam emerges from cystic structures with greater intensity than if it had passed through solid tissue and will produce louder echoes in the underlying tissue *(arrows)*.

What To Do

Shadowing (and enhancement) are mixed blessings; they give us information about the nature of an interface, but they also hide a lot of anatomy and deceive us by creating "pseudomasses." It is frequently possible to remove an offending shadow by changing the patient's position or the scan plane. When rib shadows make the liver look like a venetian blind, having the patient take deep breaths in and out will cause parts of the liver to move in and out of view in the gaps between the shadows. If the urinary bladder is well filled it will push the small bowel out of the pelvis and uncover the pelvic organs. Changing the scan plane to look under the stomach will frequently reveal the tail of the pancreas, which was obscured in a direct frontal approach. If you are imaginative and persistent in looking for good acoustic windows, you will usually be able to get around the problem of anatomy hiding in the shadows.

Pseudomasses are not hard to recognize *if you look for them*. The trick is to maintain a high degree of suspicion about any echo-poor or anechoic mass. If you are dealing with a real mass it will have a *back wall* (in addition to front and side walls). Pseudomasses, by contrast, never have a back wall. They appear to have side walls—an artifact created by the shadow—but they will not have a back wall.

A rose is a rose is a rose department: Did you notice that there seem to be two different kinds of shadow? One type, called a "clean" shadow, has sharp sides and an abrupt cut-off of echoes at the shadow-producing interface (Figure 4–2). The other type, called the "dirty" shadow, has sharp side walls, but its top edge is very irregular and it seems to contain some amorphous "clouds" of echoes (Figure 4–1). As a general—but not invariable—rule, "clean" shadows arise from tissue-bone or tissue–dense material interfaces, while "dirty" shadows arise from tissue-gas interfaces. The reason for the difference is reverberations.

REVERBERATIONS

Reverberations are the largest source of "positive" artifacts—"echoes" that are not real. Up until now we have been assuming that the ultrasound beam makes a straight, uninhibited trip to an interface in the body and back to the transducer. When it arrives back at the transducer, however, the interaction of the sound beam with the crystal is complex. A portion of the sound is absorbed by the transducer crystal and produces the small electric pulse that records the echo. The remainder, however, is reflected back into the patient. After all, the transducer–soft tissue interface constitutes a marked acoustic impedance mismatch that makes it an effective ultrasonic reflector. So the echo bounces off the transducer and makes a second trip through the patient to the interface, where it is once again reflected and returns to the transducer. At the transducer the same process is repeated: a signal is generated and what remains of the echo is reflected back into the patient for a third trip. (Of course, it is much weaker now, having been attenuated by two trips through the patient.) This process of the echo bouncing back and forth between two interfaces is known as **reverberation** and it will continue until the echo is totally exhausted by attenuation.

Each time the reverberating echo strikes the crystal it generates a signal. The scanner has no way of knowing that the signal arose from reverberation; all it knows is that the signal was received in twice the time as the first signal (or three times or four times, depending on how long the reverberation persists), and it records the signals generated by the reverberating echo

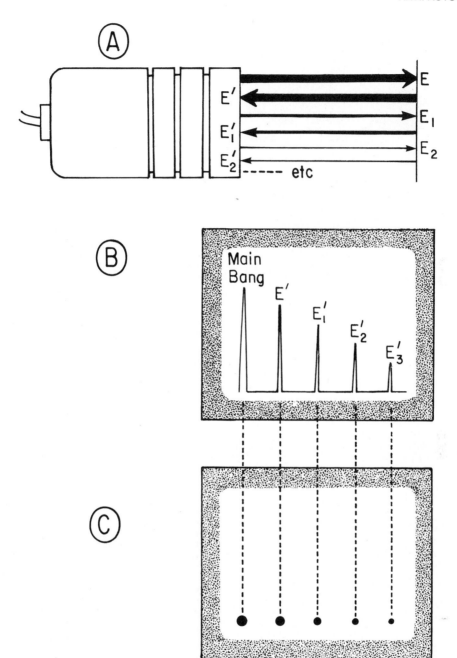

Figure 4–6. The reverberations of an echo between the transducer and an interface cause artifacts.

A. The initial pulse *(large arrow)* leaves the transducer and travels to an interface where echo E is produced. When the echo returns to the transducer it generates an electric signal, E'. The echo is reflected back into the tissue, however, and makes a second trip to the interface *(arrow)*, where another echo, E_1, is produced. When this echo returns to the transducer, it generates a second electric signal E'_1, and is again reflected into the tissue *(small arrow)*, where an additional echo, E_2, and signal, E'_2, are produced. This procedure continues until the pulse is exhausted by attenuation.

B. The A-mode presentation of the reverberation process shows one real echo signal, E', and several artifactual signals, E'_1 to E'_3. Notice that each of the artifacts occurs at a multiple of the distance to the real echo, that is, the distance from the main bang to spike E' is the same as the distance from E' to E'_1, or from E'_1 to E'_2, or E'_2 to E'_3. Because of attenuation, each succeeding spike is of smaller amplitude, and eventually the signals die out.

C. In B-mode the reverberations present as a series of dots of decreasing brightness. Only the first dot corresponds to a real echo in the patient; the others are all artifacts.

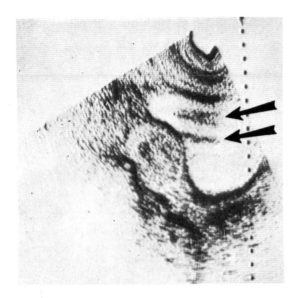

Figure 4–7. Reverberations between the body wall and the transducer face produce artifacts. In this longitudinal scan of a pelvis (notice the fibroid in the uterus) there are two prominent linear artifacts in the upper portion of the bladder *(arrows)*. It is easy to see the real echo interfaces that gave rise to these artifacts in the overlying soft tissue.

Figure 4–8. The reverberation of an echo between two internal interfaces can produce artifacts, as illustrated in lines 1 to 6. Line 1 shows a pulse passing through an interface, A, and producing echo A'. In line 2 the pulse crosses interface B, producing echo B'. (Interfaces A and B can be thought of as the front and back walls of a cyst.) When the echo B' recrosses interface A (line 3) some of it will be reflected back into the cyst. When this reflected portion encounters interface B, a second echo, B'_1, is produced (line 4). Line 5 shows that as this echo B'_1 crosses interface A again a small portion will be reflected. In line 6 echo B'_1 has returned to the transducer while the reflected portion is again encountering the back wall of the cyst, producing another echo, B'_2.

The right side of each line shows the A-mode oscilloscope tracing of these echoes. A' and B' are, of course, the true echoes from interfaces A and B; but B'_1 (and B'_2, B'_3, and the like) are artifacts.

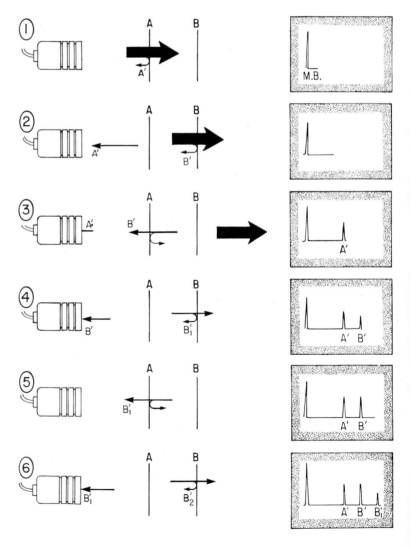

just as if they were real, placing each at a distance corresponding to the time it was received. Figure 4–6 illustrates a reverberating echo and shows how the scanner would record this in A- and B-modes. There are several things to notice about the reverberation and its artifacts.

1. Only the initial spike (or dot in B-mode) is real; it corresponds to the original echo. All the other spikes are artifacts.

2. The spikes from each of the reverberations are displayed at multiples of the distance of the interface; that is, the first artifactual spike will be twice as far from the transducer as the real echo, the second artifact will be three times this distance, and so forth.

3. Each artifact spike is smaller than the previous one because the reverberating echo is continually being attenuated by the tissue. In B-mode this is manifest as each dot being a lighter shade of gray than its predecessor.

If we examine Figure 4–6 we will be able to recognize conditions in which reverberation artifacts will be severe. First, the more reflective the interface, the more likely it is to produce reverberations. Unless an echo is strong it will not have enough amplitude to make the second journey to the interface without being completely attenuated. Echoes that arise from soft tissue–air interfaces, such as bowel gas, are loud enough to generate a significant number of reverberation artifacts. In general, echoes arising from soft tissue–soft tissue interfaces do not have sufficient amplitude to set up reverberations; however, this is not invariably true. If the interface is a large specular reflector that is located at right angles to the sound beam and is fairly close to the transducer so that there is little attenuation, reverberation artifacts can occur. The fascial planes of the anterior abdominal wall fulfill these criteria and frequently produce linear artifacts (Figure 4–7).

Second, we can see that more reverberations will be produced at high gain than at low gain. Increasing the gain gives all echoes more amplitude and means that more reverberations will survive tissue attenuation to cause artifacts.

Finally, the nearer an interface is located to the transducer, the more likely it is to cause reverberation artifacts. This is partly because there is greater attenuation of an echo from a distant interface and hence it is more likely to die out before it can reverberate. But there is another factor involved here as well. Remember that the first artifact occurs at *twice* the distance of the interface from the transducer. If the interface is at 3 cm, the first artifact occurs at 6 cm; if an interface is located 12 cm from the transducer, however, its artifact will be projected at 24 cm and will be beyond the image. Artifacts projected beyond the useful image create no problems. The use of a water delay between the transducer and the patient's skin is an effective way of increasing the distance between the transducer and interfaces and causes many reverberations to be projected beyond the useful image.

Laboratory exercise time: The full urinary bladder is an excellent subject with which to visualize the concept of reverberation artifacts. We know that the bladder does not produce any real echoes—it contains no interfaces—and hence, any "echoes" that appear in its upper portions are artifacts. Drink three beers and then go scan your bladder. Be sure to keep the transducer over the bladder—we will see why in a moment—and make a series of scans; start at low gain and slowly increase the gain as you scan. The low-gain pictures should have no "echoes" within the bladder; but as the gain is increased, reverberation artifacts will begin to appear. These will first be in the very top of the bladder; as the gain is progressively increased, they will penetrate deeper and deeper until they obscure the entire bladder, even its back wall. Next put a plastic IV bag or a Baggie full of water on your bladder and repeat the scans through the water delay. Where are the reverberations now? Finally move the transducer up to your umbilicus and try to scan the bladder from this position by angling the transducer toward your pelvis. Can you outline the bladder? Can you even find the bladder? Why are the images of the bladder so poor when it is scanned from the umbilicus? We will see in just a minute.

Internal Reverberations

We have been discussing reverberation artifacts that arise from the sound beam being reflected off the transducer face. Although these reverberations are by far the most troublesome in clinical scanning, they are not the only type of reverberations that occur. As echoes return to the transducer they encounter many interfaces, and at each there is the potential for a portion of the echo to be reflected back into the patient. Figure 4–8 illustrates how internal reverberations arise. In this schematic diagram we follow a single pulse on its journey to a cyst and back. The pulse reaches the front wall of the cyst, and an echo is produced that returns to the transducer. The pulse continues on to the back wall of the cyst, where another echo is produced. The pulse then continues on through the patient, but we will forget about it and now follow the progress of the echo produced at the back wall of the cyst. This echo starts its return journey to the transducer, but when it reaches the front wall of the cyst, a small portion of it is reflected back into the cyst. (Remember that an interface reflects sound no matter which direction the beam is traveling when it crosses it.) The portion of our echo that was not reflected back into the cyst continues on to the transducer. The reflected portion returns to the back wall of the cyst, where it is once again bounced back toward the transducer. When the reflected portion arrives at the transducer it will produce a signal that, since it was delayed on its return by the "extra" trip in the cyst, will not be recorded in the proper position, but will be located deeper in the image.

An alternative method of conceptualizing internal reverberations is to understand that small portions of echoes get delayed on their return trip to the transducer. The delays are caused by internal reflections (or reverberations) from interfaces that the echoes cross on their return trip. Any echo that is delayed in its return journey will produce an artifact, since the scanner always assumes that the echo made a direct trip to the interface and back, and places the dot in the image in a position that corresponds to a direct trip.

Because the amount of delay depends on the number of reverberations the echo undergoes before it finally returns to the transducer, and because this number is extremely variable, it is not possible to predict where the artifacts will be projected into the image (unlike reverberations from the transducer face whose artifacts are projected at multiples of the original distance). It is, therefore, extremely difficult to recognize the artifacts produced by internal reverberations (for all practical purposes they are impossible to distinguish from real echoes). Fortunately for clinical ultrasonography, the interfaces in the body do not reflect sound as effectively as the transducer face, so the percentage of echoes that produce internal reverberation artifacts is relatively small.

By this time you have figured out that gas and bone are the champion artifact producers. The acoustic impedance mismatch is so great that very high-amplitude echoes and reverberations are the rule. Even if the amount of gas is small—only a few bubbles, for instance—there will be many artifacts produced. When the sound beam encounters bowel gas, it is totally blocked; there is no way to "blast" through it by turning up the gain, and consequently there is no way to generate echoes from underlying structures. Any "echoes" that appear beyond bowel gas are artifacts, no matter how high the gain is set. At low gain there are fewer artifacts than at high gain; and this probably accounts for the common misconception that increasing the gain blasts the sound beam through gas.

Appearance of Reverberations

In Figure 4–7 we saw reverberations in their simplest and most easily recognized form— bands of "echoes" in an area where there should be no echoes. Things are not so obvious when these reverberations are projected onto the image of an organ, however. Figure 4–9 shows artifacts from the abdominal wall projected into the liver. When there are many internal reverberations the appearance can be quite variable. Figure 4–10 shows the common appearance of the left upper quadrant; bubbles of air in the stomach give rise to a complex pattern of "echoes," all of which are artifacts. Figure 4–11 shows the common appearance of the lower aorta; its lumen is cluttered and partially obscured by clouds of artifacts arising from gas in the overlying small bowel. Figure 4–12 demonstrates how artifacts from the colon can completely obscure the fundus or lower portion of the gallbladder. Figure 4–13 is a scan of the common carotid artery made with a high-resolution scanner; the artifacts in the upper portion of the vessel arise from internal reverberations in the thickened, slightly calcified arterial wall. Figure 4–14 shows low-level reverberation "echoes" in the blood vessels of the porta hepatis arising from internal reflections in the liver. (By now you should understand why it is difficult to scan the bladder when the transducer is positioned near the umbilicus.)

What To Do

After this dissertation on the plague of reverberation artifacts, you may be tempted to give

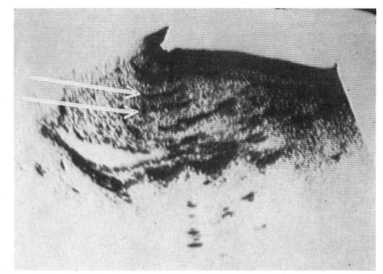

Figure 4-9. Reverberation artifacts are harder to recognize when they are projected onto normal echo-producing areas. In this longitudinal scan through the right lobe of the liver there are two linear reverberation artifacts from the overlying body wall (*white arrows*) superimposed on the normal liver echoes.

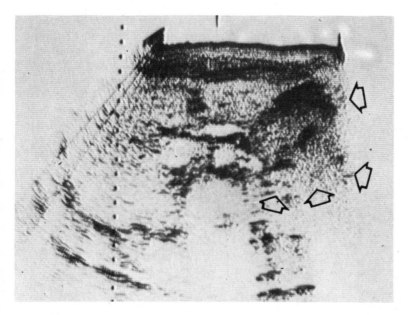

Figure 4-10. The left upper quadrant of the abdomen is frequently obscured by bowel gas artifacts. This transverse scan of a normal upper abdomen shows a typical appearance of the artifacts that arise from air in the stomach or splenic flexure of the colon (*open arrows*). No matter how little air is in the stomach, when the patient is supine this air rises to the gastric antrum, where it is in an excellent position to cause artifacts.

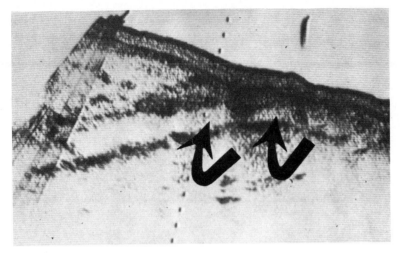

Figure 4–11. Subtle reverberation artifacts can be very difficult to recognize. In this longitudinal scan through the aorta there are several "clouds" of small echoes in the lumen of the lower aorta *(curved arrows)*. These are not real echoes; they are artifacts from small amounts of gas in the overlying bowel.

up ultrasound for ditch-digging or some other straightforward field. Have faith! Although reverberations are ever present, the sonographer can learn to recognize them and take steps to minimize their production and effect.

The first rule is *always to scan at the lowest gain compatible with a complete image.* Remember that at higher gain more reverberations will survive attenuation and appear in the image. We will discuss proper setting of the gain controls in the next chapter.

Mine is better than yours department: In the frenzied competition to see which machine can have the highest-frequency transducer, the quality of the image has sometimes suffered. Higher-frequency transducers must be operated at higher gain, and the resulting increase in artifacts frequently overshadows the small improvement in resolution. If you are

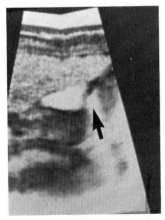

Figure 4–12. The combination of shadowing and reverberations from gas in the colon sometimes obscures the fundus of the gallbladder.

getting a lot of artifacts in the picture, try using a lower-frequency transducer at lower gain; the quality of the image will usually improve.

The next rule is to *avoid scanning in situations or areas that are prone to produce artifacts.* Because the greatest cause of artifacts is a gas–soft tissue interface, the ultrasound beam should never be allowed to pass through gas-bearing bowel if it can be avoided. For scanning the upper abdomen, the transducer should be kept over the liver as much as possible rather than scanning through the stomach or colon. When the pelvis is being scanned, the urinary bladder must be full; this lifts the small intestine out of the pelvis and permits the sound beam to reach the pelvic organs without having to traverse artifact-producing bowel gas. This process is frequently referred to as "scanning through an **acoustic window.**" This is an excellent description of an important concept: In ultrasound scanning there are "acoustic windows" and "acoustic walls"; the sound beam can "see" through the windows but not the walls. Bowel, with its ever-present gas, is a wall, and passing the beam through it is apt to produce artifacts. Soft tissue organs like the liver, the urinary bladder, and the kidneys are windows; scanning through them gives a useful picture. The good ultrasonographer will take advantage of acoustic windows.

It is not always possible to avoid scanning over gas; scans of the aorta, for instance, must be performed through bowel. Although the image often has many artifacts, it is still useful because we know what the aorta is supposed to look like and, therefore, can separate it from the artifacts. The same holds for abdominal

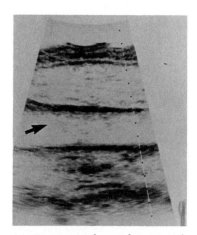

Figure 4–13. Internal reverberations from thick arterial walls can produce artifacts in the lumen of the vessel. This high-resolution image (the dots are spaced at 2.5 mm) of the common carotid artery shows a band of reverberation artifacts *(arrow)* underneath the anterior wall.

masses that are palpable; it may be possible to scan such masses through bowel because we have some idea of what we are looking for. The retroperitoneal lymph nodes are another example of a structure that can be recognized in the presence of artifacts. If, on the other hand, there is no clear idea of the type of mass that is being searched for, we must be very cautious when scanning through bowel. When a scan is made through bowel it is probably wise to verify any suspected abnormality by some other means such as physical examination, CT scan, x-ray, or isotope scan.

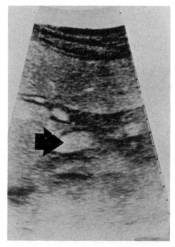

Figure 4–14. Internal reverberation artifacts are present in the vessels of the porta hepatis *(arrow)*.

EFFECTS OF TRANSDUCER FOCUS

Improvements in transducer focusing have had the paradoxical effect of producing some artifacts in the image. The most common is intensification of the beam in the focal zone. Remember in Chapter 2 we saw how focusing causes the beam to narrow in the focal zone and spread out in the near and far fields? (Consult Figure 2–11 if you were asleep when we discussed that.) As the beam is squeezed down it is also concentrated so that it is "hotter" in the focal zone than in the near and far fields. What effect will this have on the picture? As Figure 4–15 shows, this creates enhancement of the echoes in the focal zone relative to the rest of the image. It is not the enhancement that usually causes trouble, however. Rather it is the lack of enhancement in the far field, which can be mistaken for an echo-poor abnormality.

Since shadowing (and acoustic enhancement) depend upon an interface blocking (or failing to block) the sound beam, the width of the beam will determine how small an interface can produce a shadow. Consider a hypothetical sound beam that has a diameter of 3 mm at its focal point, but widens to 10 mm in the near and far fields. Suppose we pass this beam over a gallstone that is 3 mm in diameter. If the gallstone is located at the same depth as the focal point it will totally block the beam and cast a shadow. If, on the other hand, the stone is located in the near or far field where the beam is 10 mm across, only a small percentage (about 10 per cent) will be blocked and the stone will probably not cast a perceptible shadow. The point to remember is that shadowing depends not only on the reflectivity of an interface but also on its size relative to the beam width and its position relative to the focal zone. If a suspected gallstone does not cast a shadow, it may be because it is not located in the focal zone of the transducer.

A corollary to this is that the better the focus, the more pronounced the effect of shadowing and enhancement. Figure 4–16 illustrates a normal liver scanned with a finely focused beam; the narrow beam causes the portal venous branches to produce acoustic shadowing that could easily be mistaken for metastases by the unwary.

What To Do

There is no such thing as a free lunch. Improved transducers have better focus and

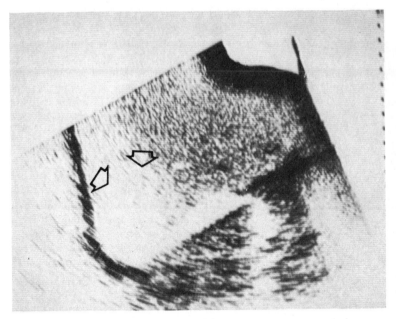

Figure 4–15. The spreading and attenuation of the beam in the far field can easily be mistaken for a mass or echo-poor lesion. The apparent "echo-poor" mass deep in the liver (*arrow*) is just an artifact due to excessive attenuation and loss of focus.

resolution, but they also magnify the differences between the focal zone and the near and far fields and accentuate the production of shadows and acoustic enhancement. The first problem can be minimized by adjusting the TCG amplifier to compensate for the increased beam intensity in the focal zone. Continued transducer improvements such as variable or electronic focusing will also reduce this artifact. The second problem requires an adjustment in the ultrasonologist's mind; he must develop a standard for what is a normal amount of shadowing with the transducer-scanner combination he is using. What is "normal" with one machine may be abnormal with another. For example, we used to call any degree of heterogeneity in the liver abnormal; now we temper that opinion, since we commonly see minor degrees of heterogeneity from enhancement by the blood vessels.

ELECTRONIC NOISE

An ultrasound scanner is a highly complex electronic device that is subject to "noise" from random electron movements. There is noise inherent in the production and reception of the echo pulse and in the display systems for presenting and photographing the image. To the extent that noise is converted to low-level "echoes" in the image, it represents a form of positive artifact. A cyst may never appear completely echo-free because low-level signals from electronic noise are superimposed on the picture. Some scanners are sensitive to low-frequency radio signals, others need a more stable power supply than is available in the hospital circuits. We sometimes get interference from the electrocautery unit in the operating room of the hospital. When the machine needs adjusting (a tune-up) the noise in the picture increases.

What To Do

Excessive noise can be a frustrating problem for which there are no easy solutions. The place to start is with the service man. Keep calling him back until the picture is satisfactory. When the machine is working well, make several representative pictures *of yourself* to keep as a standard. When you suspect the noise is getting worse repeat these scans and compare them. When you have a service call be certain the repairman does not leave until the scanner meets your "standard." If there is outside interference, it will take real detective work to ferret out the cause. Keep records of when the problems occur and try to match them with

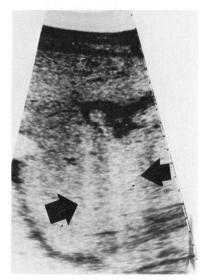

Figure 4–16. Tightly focused beams augment the effects of shadowing and acoustic enhancement. This scan of the liver was made with a 5 mm beam. There is acoustic shadowing beneath the portal vessels, which gives the liver texture a heterogeneous appearance not unlike that of metastases.

other activity in the hospital, particularly in adjoining rooms or on common power lines.

IMPERFECT ANATOMY

This is not an artifact per se, but it can be just as frustrating as all the other artifacts combined. Some patients' internal anatomy is such that it defies all attempts to scan it.

The most common cause of this problem is a small left lobe of the liver. As we shall see, the liver is the main acoustic window in abdominal scanning, and a prominent left lobe is vital to getting a good look at the pancreas and the left retroperitoneum. Most patients have nice full left lobes; there is, however, a group of people with small left lobes (this is of no clinical significance; livers, like breasts and noses, come in all sizes and shapes). When the left lobe of the liver is small, the stomach occupies not only the left upper quadrant but the central abdomen as well, and the shadow from the air it invariably contains can completely exclude the ultrasound beam. Some patients have very narrow livers that permit the transverse colon and its gas to rise up to the level of the pancreas and obscure it. Short stocky patients are frequently difficult to scan because their livers are located high up under the rib cage and are

inaccessible. The kidneys in these patients are hidden away under ribs and bowel.

Fat has a very deleterious effect on the ultrasound beam. The reasons for this are not completely clear but probably relate to the multiple interfaces that are present in lipomatous tissue and give rise to numerous small echoes and beam refraction. Excessive absorption of the sound beam may also play a role. For whatever reason, the ultrasonographer quickly learns that fat is his enemy. Slender patients are very photogenic (or sonogenic if you prefer), while obese patients are nearly impossible to scan. In very fat patients the sound beam barely makes it through the abdominal wall—on several occasions in obese patients we have had difficulty in even finding the pregnant uterus, let alone identifying the placenta or fetus. Very skinny patients are no bargain either. For reasons that elude us, the quality of the scan in asthenic patients is often surprisingly poor (maybe a little fat is necessary to outline the organ boundaries).

What To Do

Keep a stiff upper lip. There is nothing you can do about the weight or internal make-up of your patients. The popular ultrasound expression for these scanning situations is "excessive bowel gas." This is a good descriptive term but it is somewhat misleading, since it implies that the phenomenon is transient and that if the patient is brought back another day (or given a special diet or antiflatulants or whatever) you will be able to make a good scan. The idea is attractive but, in our experience, does not work. The real cause of "excessive bowel gas" is imperfect internal anatomy that does not provide an adequate acoustic window for viewing the abdomen. This anatomy is not going to be altered. The most skilled ultrasonographer in the world cannot generate good pictures in a very obese patient, and even the rank beginner will make beautiful images in a Miss America. The trick is to get the most information possible, given the limits imposed by the body habitus of the patient. The truly skillful ultrasonographer will be able to scrape together a diagnostic examination in many cases in which the less experienced will be forced to punt. In the end, though, if you cannot see clearly, be honest and say so in the report. The referring physician and the patient are depending on your information and expect you to be accurate.

BIBLIOGRAPHY

Sommer, F. G., Filly, R. A., and Minton, M. J.: Acoustic shadowing due to refractive and reflective effects. *American Journal of Roentgenology 132*:973 (1979).
(This article is somewhat technical but has a nice discussion and illustrations of various shadowing and enhancement phenomena.)

Jaffe, C. C., and Taylor, K. J. W.: The clinical impact of ultrasonic beam focusing patterns. *Radiology 131*:469 (1979).
(Further discussion of the artifacts created by beam focusing. It is alarming that a large percentage of those doing ultrasound are still unaware of this problem.)

Robinson, D. E., Wilson, L. S., and Kossoff, G.: Shadowing and enhancement in ultrasonic echograms by reflection and refraction. *Journal of Clinical Ultrasound 9*:181 (1981).
(For you physics freaks here is a more sophisticated explanation of shadowing artifacts.)

Chapter 5

GENERAL SCANNING TECHNIQUES

Have you ever taken piano lessons? Dancing lessons? Perhaps you remember physical education classes in school in which, for what seemed like an interminable amount of time, you were forced to practice exercises, or "fundamentals" as they were called? Our personal experience was with piano lessons. Half of every lesson and half of every practice session were devoted to technical exercises—scales, arpeggios, finger exercises, and the like. The reasoning behind this drudgery escaped us at the time. The teacher said that it was important to learn the technique of piano playing through exercises; they could be practiced over and over until perfected, and while this made the exercise itself unpleasant, it enabled us eventually to acquire the technique to play Chopin. Now, years later, most of this technique has been forgotten, and today when we try to play Chopin it is tough. Each difficult passage must be struggled over and painstakingly worked out; by the time we are technically able to play the piece we hate it because it was so much work.

Ultrasound scanning is somewhat the same. A certain amount of technical expertise is required to produce clinically useful images; until this technique is mastered scanning is a hassle. The ultrasonographer must spend so much time and effort trying to produce a good picture (fiddling with the dials, trying to get the patient in a good position, loading the camera, dropping the oil can) that he is unable to concentrate on the real business at hand, which is making a diagnosis or answering a clinical question. Fortunately, the technique of scanning is not hard to acquire, particularly with real-time scanners, and if the beginner spends some time mastering it, he will soon come to the point at which he has no difficulty obtaining diagnostically useful information. The material in this chapter rep-

resents the scales and arpeggios of scanning—the "fundamentals." As such, it is the most important part of the entire text; once the fundamentals are mastered, the ultrasonographer is equipped to perform good examinations and to alter and expand his technique to cope with unusual and difficult scanning situations.

PREPARATION AND SUPPLIES

Because ultrasound scanning involves considerable cooperation between patient and sonographer, it is important not only that the patient be comfortable but also that he sense a feeling of professionalism and competence about the sonographer and the examination process. Creating this atmosphere requires prior preparation and planning.

It goes without saying that the examining room should be neat and tidy, and that items you will need during the examination—coupling agent, film cassettes, towels, and the like—should be close at hand. The examination table should be freshly made up with clean sheets and a fluffed-up pillow. Be sure to have extra sheets and a blanket; remember the patient does not have much on and is often not feeling up to par. Have a step handy so that he can climb onto the table easily, and provide a space for personal items such as a purse or glasses. While getting the patient into the room and onto the examining table, explain what the procedure will involve, stressing that it is: (1) comfortable, (2) safe, (3) will not last long, and (4) requires the patient's help in order to get good results.

The transducer must be in close contact with the patient's skin so that there is minimum attenuation of the sound beam. It is particularly important to exclude air (remember, we saw in Chapter 1 that air will completely block the beam). Either mineral oil or an aqueous gel is used to provide this good contact between the skin and transducer. Mineral oil does not dry out, resists being wiped away by the transducer, and is a good lubricant between the transducer and skin. Its only disadvantage is the messiness; it is difficult to wipe off and soils clothing. Aqueous gels are easy to clean up and do not damage clothing, but they tend to dry out and are rather easily wiped away by the transducer. They do not lubricate as well as oil and are much more expensive. Aqueous gels, however, are also more viscous than oil and can provide acoustic coupling over very rough surfaces (when there is lots of body hair, for instance) where oil sometimes fails. We use mineral oil for the bulk of our scanning but keep a small amount of gel on hand for special occasions. The oil is purchased in bulk and dispensed from a plastic squeeze bottle (the kind that is used for ketchup and mustard). If you really want to go first class you can buy a baby bottle warmer to keep the oil at body temperature, but we just warn the patient that the oil will be "a little cold." Some instruments can only be used with a specific coupling agent, so it is worthwhile to check with the technical specialist from the company when you first install a new machine so that you do not harm it inadvertently.

The important thing to remember about coupling agents is to use enough. As scanning progresses, the oil or gel is wiped away by the transducer, and acoustic coupling decreases. The change in the picture is subtle; but because of the slowly increasing attenuation, the weaker echoes die out and the picture quality fades away. Failure to use enough coupling agent is one of the most common errors we find in beginning ultrasonographers. From the start, then, we urge you to use lots of oil and reapply it liberally throughout the scan; if the picture quality starts to deteriorate, the first thing to do is to add more oil.

No matter how carefully we try to avoid it during examination, oil seems to get everywhere and on everything; therefore, we ask our patients to undress and put on examining gowns before the examination—everything but shoes, socks, and bras must go. (Resist the temptation to spare underpants or pantyhose; they will inevitably get soiled.) Having the patient undress is also important to the ultrasonographer because it makes available many potential acoustic windows that might otherwise be covered by clothing.

Finally, be sure to look over the requisition and learn something about the patient *before* you bring him into the room; this will do wonders in creating the atmosphere of professionalism and individual concern that is so important for good rapport. It is also vital in structuring the subsequent examination. As we shall see, a good ultrasound examination is not a mindless picture-taking expedition; rather, it is a planned study of individual organs and areas to delineate any anatomic abnormalities and shed some light (? sound) on the cause of the patient's symptoms. Usually the necessary information is available on the requisition. If not, it may be helpful to look at the patient's chart (assuming you can read the handwriting).

Platitudes department: How many times have you heard the pious admonition, "review the patient's chart," implying that the sonographer should pore over every temperature graph, lab result, and x-ray report as if he were a hungry malpractice attorney looking for something to pounce upon? Reading a chart like this is a mind-numbing experience, particularly in a teaching hospital, and it is not at all what we mean. The sonographer's goal in chart review is to answer three basic questions: (1) What are the patient's symptoms? (2) What diseases are under consideration? (3) What specific questions does the referring doctor want answered? Question 1 is usually answered by the first line on the first page, which is known as the "chief complaint." The answer to question 2 is at the end of the initial work-up and is usually labeled "Impression" or "Differential Diagnosis." Immediately following this should appear "Plan," in which the doctor discusses his plan of attack, listing the examinations and treatments he wants and why. The "plan" usually answers question 3. This is idealized, of course. More often than not, you will not be able to get all the information you would like. Rather than plowing willy-nilly through the chart, it is much faster (and more informative) to ask the patient yourself as you are bringing him into the room: "I know you have already told Dr. Feelgood about your problem, but it is always helpful if we can hear about it directly from you. Tell me what is bothering you and why you think the doctor wanted you to have this ultrasound scan."

SCANNING MOTIONS

Now that the patient is on the table and well greased, it is time to take the transducer in hand and make a scan. By the time you read this, most manual scanners will be on their way to a well-deserved place of honor in the Ultrasound Hall of Fame and you will be using a real-time scanner for your examinations. As we shall see in a moment, not only is real-time scanning much, much easier to do, it is also faster and more accurate as well. Because there are still some manual static scanners around, however, the skillful sonographer should know how to operate them as well as a real-time machine. In using a manual scanner there are four basic scanning motions: simple, sector, compound, and single pass.

Simple scanning involves moving the transducer in a straight line across the skin without angling the sound beam, as illustrated in Figure 5–1. With the simple scan the sound beam passes over each reflector only once and strikes each interface at only one angle. This is the same scanning motion used by a rectilinear radioisotope scanner or the pick-up head of a tape recorder. (In the latter case it is the tape

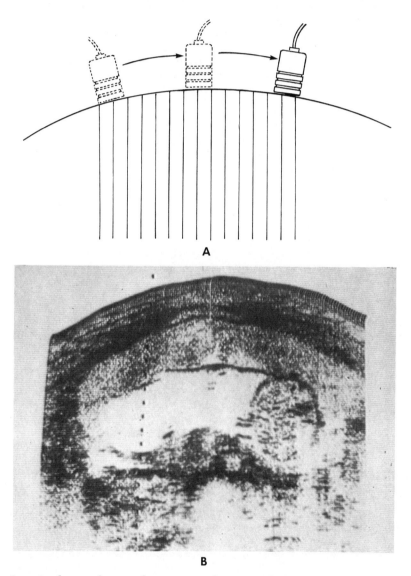

A

B

Figure 5–1. In a *simple* scan the transducer is moved in a straight line across the abdomen.

A. Diagrammatic representation of a simple scan. The sound beam passes over each interface only once and strikes each reflector at only one angle.

B. A simple scan of a pregnant uterus.

rather than the head that is moving, but the scanning effect is the same.)

Sector scanning involves pivoting the transducer so that the sound beam is rotated about the transducer face, as illustrated in Figure 5–2. The pattern of the sound beam resembles a wedge of pie (known in mathematical circles as

a "sector"). This is the type of scanning motion our eyes use as they read a line of print; they start at the left and pivot across the line to the right. Radar also uses a sector scanning motion; we have all seen the radarscope at an airport, rotating as it scans the sky. In sector scanning, as in simple scanning, the sound beam passes

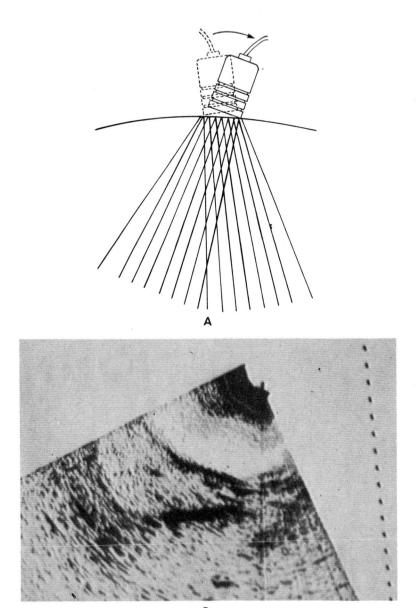

A

B

Figure 5–2. When the transducer is pivoted about its face a *sector* scan is produced.

A. Diagrammatic representation of a sector scan. The sound beam passes over each interface only once and strikes each reflector at only one angle.

B. A sector scan of a normal female pelvis.

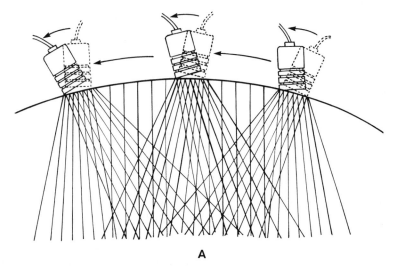

A

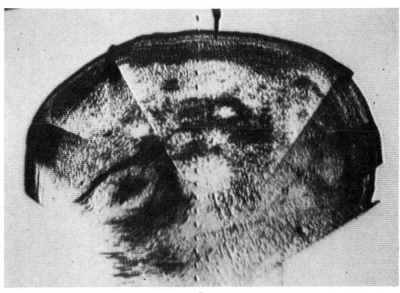

B

Figure 5–3. When the transducer is moved so that the sound beam passes over interfaces more than once and strikes reflectors from more than one angle, a *compound* scan is produced.

A. Diagrammatic representation of a compound scan.

B. A compound scan of the upper abdomen.

over each reflector only once and strikes each interface at only one angle.

Compound scanning is sometimes described as a combination of simple and sector scanning, but this is a poor definition. We prefer to consider compound scanning as any scan motion that causes the sound beam to pass over a reflector more than once or causes the beam to strike the interface from more than one angle. Obviously there are many scanning motions that fit this definition. The one most frequently used is the sliding, rocking motion illustrated in

Figure 5–3. Compound scanning is the way our eyes evaluate a new car (or an attractive member of the opposite sex), peering up, down, from side to side, and all around. This technique was developed in the early days of ultrasound for bi-stable scanning. Bi-stable scanners were primarily interested in specular echoes—those loud reflections from organ boundaries. Because specular reflections are angle-dependent, it was important that the sound beam strike each interface from several different angles so that the loudest echo was received; it did not matter that the beam passed through some interfaces several times, distorting the relative amplitudes of the echoes. The introduction of the gray scale in the mid-1970's changed things. In gray-scale scanning we are interested primarily in the small, non-angle-dependent, non-specular echoes and we want to maintain the correct amplitude relationship between them. For this reason compound scanning is not a suitable technique with gray-scale imaging.

The correct scanning motion for gray-scale is what we call the **single pass scan**; a combination of simple and sector scanning. How the transducer is moved is not especially important as long as two conditions are met: The transducer must always remain over an "acoustic window," and the sound beam should not pass over any interface more than once.

We discussed the importance of the acoustic window in Chapter 4, and there is no need for further exposition on that point. We want to be certain, however, that everyone understands the importance of the second point—the sound beam should not pass over an interface more than once. The value of gray-scale scanning rests in its ability to display the relative amplitudes of the echo interfaces; this is what produces the shades of gray and gives the image texture. It is through this texture that the ultrasonographer arrives at a diagnostic decision. For the texture, or gray scale, to have meaning, each interface must be scanned only one time; each interface gets one chance to produce an echo. If the sound beam passes over interface A once and over interface B twice we can see that, aside from the inherent difference in the two interfaces, B will have a greater chance to produce an echo than A. If interface C is scanned five times, it will almost certainly produce a darker echo than if it were scanned only once.

Manufacturers have tried to minimize this effect with circuits to prevent overwriting of the display. These circuits compensate only partially, however; they can do nothing to affect the echo production and they cannot eliminate the problem, as is illustrated in Figure 5–4. Good scanning technique requires "equality of opportunity"—that is, every interface should have the same opportunity to produce an echo as its neighbor; this is possible only if the sound beam is passed over each interface once and once only.

There are many ways to produce a single pass scan—usually it involves a sort of sliding sector motion. The transducer is initially aimed at one side of the patient and sectored until it is oriented approximately vertically; it is then moved over the skin surface until the end of the acoustic window is reached. The transducer is not moved off the window; instead it is again sectored. Figure 5–5 shows the progression of a single pass scan. This process is somewhat difficult to describe, and the best way to get a feel for it is to practice some scans—you will quickly get the knack. The entire scan motion should consist of a single smooth sweep. The hardest part is staying over the acoustic window, but if you watch the image as it is built up on the TV screen, you will be able to tell when the transducer reaches the edge of the window. (There is no harm in moving off the window as long as you realize the limited value of the resulting image.)

Real-time scanners move the beam automatically, so we need not worry about all this stuff. They all make a single pass motion, and the only thing the sonographer must do is aim them. The "sector-scanner" type of machine has a small scan line at the skin surface and is easy to keep over an acoustic window. The "wide-field" type of machine has a longer scan line, and frequently some of the image will extend past the acoustic window. This is no problem for diagnosis—just ignore the portion of the scan that was not made through the window—but it does make the overall picture seem messier. (The beauty of the picture is not really important, however; what counts is the quality of the diagnosis.)

Finally, a word about patient breathing. The three biggest problems confronting the sonographer are: (1) finding an acoustic window, (2) finding an acoustic window, and (3) finding an acoustic window. The liver and spleen are the main acoustic windows into the abdomen (what is the acoustic window for the pelvis?). Some or all of these organs are hidden up under the rib cage, and by controlling the patient's respiration you can bring different areas into view. In later chapters we shall discuss specific ways of seeing different areas, but one general rule is useful to keep in mind: It is almost always easier to see the upper abdomen when the patient is holding his breath in deep inspiration. This brings more of the liver and spleen out from under the ribs and widens the acoustic window.

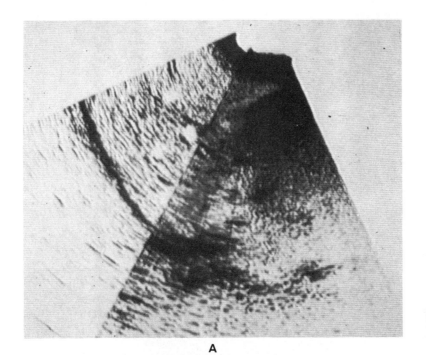

A

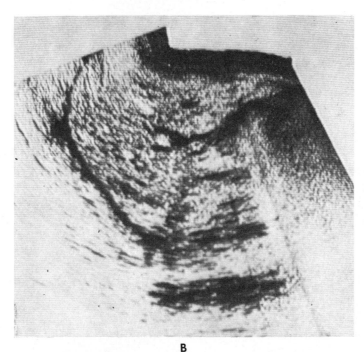

B

Figure 5–4. Passing the sound beam over an interface more than once distorts the gray scale.

A. A longitudinal scan through the right lobe of the liver. The sound beam was started on the left and swept across the liver to the right and then swept halfway back; the interfaces on the right half of the picture are darker than those on the left, and there is an artifactual boundary in the liver.

B. The same scan as in *A*, except that the sound beam was passed over the liver only once. The echoes have the same intensity and it is easy to see that the liver is normal.

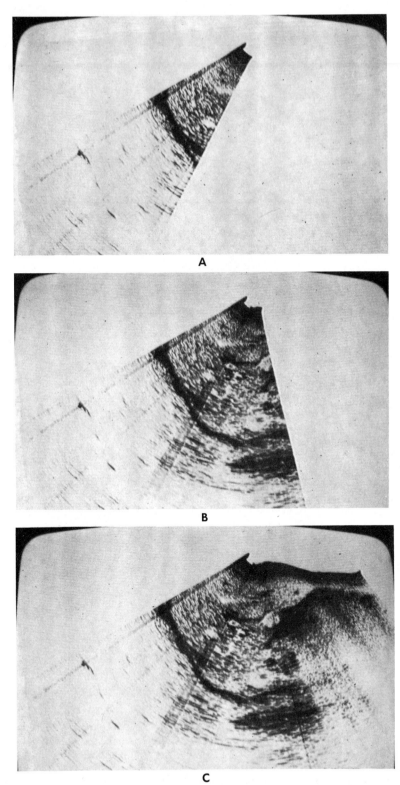

A

B

C

Figure 5–5. Gray-scale scanning requires a *single pass* technique. The buildup of a single pass scan is shown in pictures *A*, *B*, and *C*; this is a longitudinal scan through the right lobe of the liver.

SCANNER CONTROLS

The best scanning technique in the world will be worthless if the scanner is not properly adjusted. Although at first glance the scanning console may appear quite forbidding, there are actually very few adjustments to be made. Most of those extra knobs are put there to make the machine seem "more sophisticated" than its competitors. They are known in the trade as "bells and whistles"; and, while often providing minor conveniences, they are not essential for performing quality scans. The situation is similar with modern stereo equipment. There are, however, two very important controls that require continuous monitoring and adjustment: the TCG and the gain.

The purpose of **TCG** (Time Compensated Gain) is to give a balanced picture; it is correctly adjusted when the density of echoes is the same throughout the image. If the echoes in the near field are darker than those in the far field, the TCG is too low. If the far-field echoes are darker than the near-field ones, the TCG is too high. Every TCG control has some kind of scale associated with it, and in the past some authors and manufacturers have given "recommendations" as to where the TCG should be set for different types of examinations. In general these recommendations are not useful. There is no way to predict in any particular circumstance what amount of TCG will be needed, because this depends largely on the characteristics of the transducer and the type of tissue through which the beam is traveling. *The only correct way to adjust this control in every scanning situation is by eye.* If the far-field echoes are weak, turn up the TCG; if the near field is washed out, turn it down.

As shown in Figure 5–6, the goal is uniform echo density throughout the picture. The situation is analogous to adjusting the "balance" control on a stereo system: You listen and turn the knob until the sound is right. Do the same with the TCG: Look at the picture and adjust the control until the echoes are "balanced" throughout the image.

Know your machine department: Some scanners have a single TCG control, while others have a series of controls. The same principles apply in either circumstance. The multiple controls give greater flexibility in balancing the echo density but are less convenient to use.

At the beginning of every scan the TCG must be adjusted to fit that patient. Place the scanner over the right lobe of the liver, just below the costal margin, and make an image through the deepest part of the right lobe and the dia-

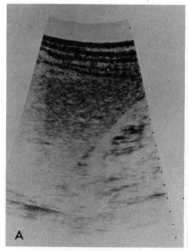 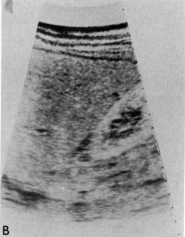

Figure 5–6. The time compensated gain (TCG) must be adjusted to give a balanced appearance to the image.

A. The TCG is set too low; echoes in the near field are louder than those in the far field.

B. The TCG is correctly adjusted and the echoes are uniform throughout the image.

phragm. Now adjust the TCG until all the echoes in the liver—those in the near, middle, and far fields—are the same shade of gray. That is all there is to it. It takes only 15 seconds; but if you skip this adjustment, all your images will be poor, and the examination will be much more difficult.

Once the TCG is adjusted, the **gain** must be set. (For convenience we shall assume that all machines have a single gain control; this may be labeled "gain" or "output" or "sensitivity"— consult the instruction manual of your scanner to find out which. If there is more than one gain control, as was common in older scanners, adjustments should be made in only one.) The gain determines the overall density of the picture. Continuing our analogy with a stereo system, if the TCG is the "balance," the gain is the "volume"; increasing it raises the strength of all the echoes uniformly.

With gray-scale scanning we want to display every echo; we will separate them on the basis of their relative amplitudes. Therefore, the gain should be adjusted so that echoes are received from all organs and tissues. The only echoless areas on the scan should be fluid-filled structures such as the gallbladder, urinary bladder, aorta, amniotic cavity, and cysts. *Solid tissues should never be echo-free; if they are the gain is set too low.* This is by far the most common error in setting the scanner controls. Almost all beginning ultrasonographers scan at too low a gain, producing a light gray liver and echo-free kidneys. Echoes that are not displayed are useless for diagnostic purposes. The main ad-

vantage of a gray-scale scanner is its ability to record all echoes on a single scan; if the gain is so low that some echoes are not recorded, much of the value of the gray scale is lost. When the gain is properly set, the liver and placenta should be medium to dark gray, and the kidneys and spleen should be light gray. Of course the capsules of the liver and kidneys and the walls of major vessels will appear very dense, since these tissues reflect large specular echoes, many times the magnitude of the parenchymal echoes.

Unfortunately, as the gain is increased, artifacts increase, and thus there is a point of diminishing return; that is, at some point a further increase in gain results in the generation of more artifacts than real echoes. The ultrasonographer's job is to find that point and set the gain control so that the image displays the maximum number of real echoes with a minimum of artifacts. This takes skill. Because it is easier to recognize when the gain is set too low than when it is too high, the scan should be started at relatively low gain and the level increased until the proper point is found. Figure 5–7 shows examples of correct and incorrect gain settings.

Always keep in mind the relationship between transducer frequency and attenuation. In Chapter 2 we saw that because of attenuation, high frequencies cannot penetrate to deeper tissue depths. All the gain in the world will not display an echo that was never received. In large patients in whom you are having trouble seeing the lower portions of the liver or kidneys

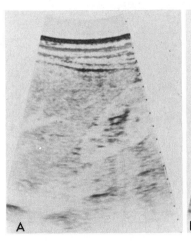
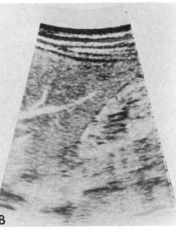

A   B

Figure 5–7. The gain must be set high enough for all solid tissues to produce echoes.

A. The gain is too low; there are very few echoes in the renal cortex.

B. The gain has been increased to the proper level.

it is often useful to change to a *lower*-frequency transducer; higher resolution is not worth anything if you can not receive the echo.

The **zoom** or **expansion** control can be useful. In this mode the image is enlarged so that a portion of the scan can be seen in greater detail. In some instruments this is done electronically, in others optically. The end result is that some of the limitation in resolution of the TV system can be overcome. When an image is expanded, the loss of resolution is reduced. This is of particular benefit when measuring a structure such as the bile duct or a small fetal head. Use the zoom or expansion controls so that the area you are scanning occupies as much of the display screen as possible. Interfaces can then be more easily separated.

Finally a word about **image processing**. As we saw in Chapter 3, most new scanners offer some type of image processing, the effect of which is to change the contrast *in the image*. This should be distinguished from the "contrast" control on the TV monitor. As we shall see in a moment, the TV contrast control does not affect the contrast *in the image*. Using the image processing controls to alter image contrast may be useful, particularly when looking for subtle differences in tissue texture. We have found this helpful in evaluating the liver for metastases and the thyroid for small lesions.

Unlike TCG and gain, image processing is a very subjective business; no three people can agree on what makes the image better or worse. Probably the best way to utilize these controls is to freeze a nice image of a portion of the liver, right kidney, and pancreas on the screen and then photograph it, using each of the available processing options. Get everyone in the lab together and have them rank each processing option (by *secret* ballot): They should vote not only for their favorite but also for the one they think is most "contrasty" (greatest variation between lowest-level and highest-level echoes) and the one they feel is least "contrasty." There will probably be general agreement in the most and least contrast categories and disagreement about the favorite. Through negotiation, threats, passive resistance, or whatever, your laboratory should agree on a favorite and use it as "standard" image processing for all general scanning.

We believe that it is important that everyone's eye become adjusted to a standard appearance of the abdomen, and this can be done only if all the scans are performed with the same image processing. This allows you to become familiar with the normal and abnormal textures of the various organs and the relationship between them. Never use the alternative processing options by themselves; rather, utilize them in conjunction with the standard processing to give you a different look at the same area. Figure 5–8 compares the effect of high-contrast image processing with our standard processing in a patient with liver metastases. Image processing must be used cautiously. While it may bring out subtle textural abnormalities, it may also create the appearance

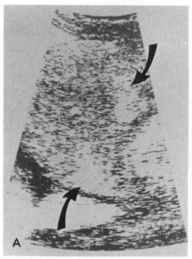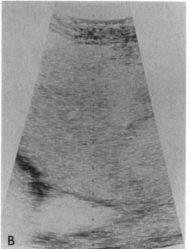

***Figure* 5–8.** Post-image processing can sometimes enhance subtle textural differences.

A. High-contrast image processing shows two lesions in the right lobe of the liver *(arrow)*.

B. The lesions are much less obvious with standard image processing.

of abnormalities where they do not exist. Always be conservative; use image processing options only as small pieces of extra information to be added to the main data generated by the standard processing.

HARD COPY

In days gone by several media were used to make a permanent record—"hard copy"—of the images; these included Polaroid film, roll film, heat-sensitive paper, sheet film, and videotape. As we learned in Chapter 3, only sheet film and videotape are widely used today. Of these, we much prefer sheet film and use videotape only to record bits of interesting cases for our teaching files. In our hands reviewing scans on videotape for the purpose of making a diagnosis has not been satisfactory; the picture changes, but we don't know where the transducer was located or how it was moved, and so we are continually lost. If scans must be performed when the ultrasonologist is unavailable (a bad practice that will inevitably get you in trouble) it may be useful to record some portions on videotape for later review by the physician.

Silver cloud–dark lining department: Film cameras come in two types: (1) a free-standing unit separate from the scanner and usually adaptable to any scanner and (2) an integral part of the scanner itself. A disadvantage of sheet film cameras is the rapacious pricing policy of the manufacturers. Eight or ten thousand dollars seems like a lot of green for a TV monitor, cheap shutter, lens, and phototimer. For instance, a standard 35 mm camera is much more sophisticated at a fraction of the price. One satisfactory compromise we have used is a manual sheet film adapter that fits on the Polaroid camera supplied with the machine. It requires the ultrasonographer to remember to change the film position, because it is not automatic, but costs less than a tenth of the price of the fancier version.

Some manufacturers are offering videodisc options as a means of making hard copy. The discs do not seem to offer any advantages over sheet film at the present time and they have one major disadvantage: They must be "played" through the scanner, and only one image can be viewed at a time. Sheet film can be flipped onto the nearest view box and can be projected easily at conferences. As image processing becomes more sophisticated, discs may find a role

as a means of storing raw data for after-the-fact image processing.

Regardless of which type of camera you choose, the viewing and hard copy TV monitors must be adjusted carefully so that the pictures come out looking like the image you saw during the scan. Once these adjustments have been made they should not be altered, come hell or high water.

Begin by adjusting the *viewing* monitor controls (the "brightness" and "contrast" knobs on the monitor itself) so that everybody thinks the picture is good. Use your "standard" image processing when making this adjustment and be certain the settings are good for all the organs, not just the liver and right kidney. Once they are set, *do not touch these controls again* (we have even resorted to removing the knobs from the monitors).

Now make a nice scan of a portion of the liver, right kidney, and pancreas with proper TCG and gain settings. Freeze this image on the screen and make a series of hard copy pictures of it while adjusting the controls (brightness and contrast) on the *hard copy* monitor. Your goal is to set these controls so that the hard copy picture looks exactly like the image on the screen. We mean *exactly*. Be very fussy here and take your time fine tuning these settings. It will probably take several sheets of film, many trips to the darkroom, and an hour of your time, but it will be worth it. After all, you will be spending many hours scanning and take thousands of pictures; you want the pictures not only to look good but also to look *like* the image you saw on the viewing screen. (We have no sympathy for those who lament that "it looked beautiful on the screen, but the hard copy is lousy." The only reason hard copy is lousy is because no one took the time to adjust the monitors properly.) Of course, if any of the controls on *either* the viewing *or* the hard copy monitor are changed, the whole process must be repeated because the pictures will no longer look like the image on the viewing screen.

It is also important to keep a record of the machine performance by regularly scanning and photographing a laboratory "test object." We do not mean a phantom or the AIUM test object; we mean a real live abdomen. Find the person in your department with the most photogenic abdomen and once a week make a scan of his liver, right kidney, and pancreas. If there is any loss of picture quality compared with the previous week's scan you will need to readjust the monitor controls. If these adjustments cannot restore the picture quality, then it is time for a service call. Do not let the service man leave until he has the machine producing a good-quality scan of your "test object." It is important to use the same person for a "test object" each time. Remember there is far more difference between individual abdomens than between different machines or even the same machine in different stages of adjustment.

With trepidation we dip our toe in the roiling waters of the black-on-white versus white-on-black image controversy. You will notice that we scan with black dots on a white background. We have tried it both ways, and everyone in our department prefers this format; we think it is easier to appreciate differences in gray scale this way. We agree it makes the picture seem a bit "noisier" than with the white-dot, black-background display. We also have no objective proof that this format is superior. In spite of claims to the contrary, we have not been convinced that those ultrasonologists who recommend the white-on-black method have objective proof of its superiority either. The whole business is subjective and not really worthy of prolonged discussion. "You pays your money and takes your choice." Once you have decided and have adjusted your scanner and camera to one format, you cannot change by simply flipping the "invert" switch. You will also have to recalibrate both the viewing and hard copy monitors.

THE PICTURE-ORIENTED EXAMINATION

In the past ultrasound has been a "picture-oriented" procedure; that is, most examinations were conducted in a manner analogous to conventional x-ray or CT imaging. The actual scanning was performed to collect a series of pictures that were then viewed by ultrasonologists who, on the basis of these pictures, formulated a diagnostic impression. With this type of examination it was obviously necessary to have some scanning coordinates for labeling the pictures so that everyone who looked at them would know exactly how and where in the patient they were performed. The development of real time and improved resolution of ultrasound scanners have rendered this "picture-oriented" scanning technique obsolete (we shall go into the reasons for this in a moment). We

no longer use, nor recommend the use of, scanning coordinates based on the external anatomy of the patient (such as "crests +2," or "lateral +3"). For those sonographers or ultrasonologists who still prefer to use this system, a standard scanning coordinate nomenclature has been approved by the American Institute of Ultrasound in Medicine and is obtainable by writing to their office in Washington, D.C.

What do we have against the traditional "picture-oriented" method of scanning? Well, nothing personal. In fact, this was a very useful method of scanning when ultrasound machines had fairly limited resolution and thick scanning slices; and it was also well suited to scanning with manual static instruments when it was difficult to change the scan plane and most scans were performed in a relatively standardized fashion. The emergence of small, mobile, hand-held real-time scanners has created tremendous flexibility and variability in scanning planes. It is virtually impossible to devise a scanning coordinate system that could accurately and easily represent the wide variety of planes used in a modern scan. Similarly, as resolution has improved, the thickness of the scan slice has been drastically reduced; a well-focused modern scanner produces a section with a thickness of 3 to 5 mm. The improved resolution and slice thickness reduction has created a new problem for the sonographer that we call "sampling error."

What do the Gallup Poll and a tomographic imaging procedure (such as ultrasound) have in common? The answer: they are both "sampling," or "polling," processes.

Left field department: You are probably thinking a better question would be "what does all of this have to do with ultrasound?" Bear with us for a moment.

A sampling, or polling, process is one in which small bits of information are collected from a much larger population or area under study. These sample data are then analyzed, and a conclusion is drawn. It is then assumed that this conclusion, based on the small sample of data, can be applied to the larger population or area from which the sample data were drawn. Most of the time this process works well because, in general, a sample will truly represent the larger population from which it is drawn. Unfortunately, occasionally the sample selected for study does not truly represent the general area or population and an erroneous conclusion is reached (we are all familiar with the occasional mistakes of the Gallup Poll.) The point is not that the sampling process is invalid; rather it is to be expected that occasionally this process will make errors because of an inappropriate sample.

Ultrasound is a sampling process. Each ultrasound image contains only a tiny amount of the total information available in the body. Furthermore, as improved resolution narrows the width of the scan slice, the size of the sample information in any single image is also reduced. As the size of the sample is reduced, the likelihood of a sampling error is increased. Figure 5–9 shows how this concept can be applied to ultrasound scanning. The patient illustrated has a tiny 3 mm gallstone in the gallbladder. The picture in 5–9A shows this tiny gallstone. Figure 5–9B is a nearly identical image; the only difference is that it was made 5 mm to the right of picture 5–9A. The tiny gallstone is not seen in this picture because it is not in the scan plane. Now consider which image you are more likely to obtain when you scan this patient's gallbladder. There will be many more potential scan planes that do not contain the tiny gallstone than do contain it. This means that on any *single* scan the sonographer is more likely to get an incorrect sample (Figure 5–9B) than a true one (Figure 5–9A). Because of this sampling error, the sonographer could incorrectly conclude that the gallbladder was normal. He would have made a diagnostic error, not because of any deficiency on his part, but because he was a victim of sampling error.

Figure 5–9 is a particularly dramatic example of sampling error, but you can understand how the same process goes on in all organs and all areas of the body. The ultrasonologist is always formulating a diagnostic decision based upon images that represent a small "sample" of the patient. As such, he will always be a potential victim for sampling error. Moreover, the smaller the potential lesion or abnormality, the more likely it is to be missed in a sampling process.

What can we do about sampling error? The only way to reduce the problem is to increase the size of the sample; as the sample size is increased, the likelihood that it will be representative of the patient will also increase. This concept will not win a Nobel Prize, but it is obvious that if we make more pictures and look at more images we will have a better idea of what is going on. The problem comes in implementation. If our scan slice thickness is 3 mm

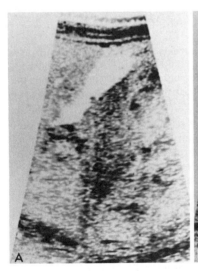 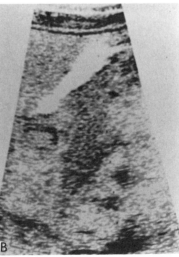

Figure 5–9. Each ultrasound image is actually a very thin tomographic "slice" of anatomy. Small lesions may be missed unless large numbers of images are examined.

A. A scan through the gallbladder demonstrates a tiny gallstone casting a small shadow.

B. A scan made 5 mm on either side of *A* gives no indication of the stone; this image would lead us to the erroneous conclusion that the gallbladder was normal.

and we wish to scan an organ such as the liver, which has dimensions of 15 by 20 cm, it would require 50 to 100 static pictures to give good coverage of this organ alone. Collecting so many pictures is clearly not practical with a manual static scanner. It is, however, no problem with a real-time scanner. These machines make between 12 and 30 pictures per second, and it is possible to collect literally hundreds of images in a minute of scanning. A real-time scanner can be "panned" back and forth across a gallbladder such as the one in Figure 5–9, sampling hundreds of sections, and the sonographer will not risk missing the scan plane that contains the small gallstone.

Real-time scanners have another great advantage over manual static scanners in addition to their ability to reduce sampling error. This is the concept of the scan plane *flexibility* we discussed earlier. Remember that the greatest difficulty in producing an ultrasound picture is finding an acoustic window that will allow the sound beam to reach the organ of interest. Many of the best acoustic windows are not available in the standard scan planes used in manual scanning. In later chapters we shall see how some areas of the body, such as the tail of the pancreas or the common bile duct, are best seen by using steeply angled and unconventional scanning planes. We shall also see that it is not always possible to predict the best scan plane for showing an individual organ or area of interest; frequently the sonographer must improvise by trying a variety of different acoustic windows and scan angles. The freely mobile real-time scanner makes it easy to explore all these possibilities, while the fixed arm system of the manual scanner limits the views that are available.

We have gone on at some length about the "philosophy" of ultrasound scanning because it is important that everyone who performs and interprets ultrasound examinations have knowledge and understanding of this area. Many of the diagnostic errors that occur in scanning result from failure to acknowledge the limitations of the scanning process and blind adherence to the concept that "it is all in the pictures." Perhaps we are so zealous because we ourselves used to suffer from this misconception. We used to conduct picture-oriented examinations and had faith that we were truly sampling the patient. We clung to tried-and-true scan planes and resigned ourselves to the tail of the pancreas being an area that was not

normally seen on ultrasound scans. We used to place an imaginary checkerboard on the patient's abdomen and conduct scans at fixed intervals based on the external anatomy, trusting that good karma would somehow make an appropriate acoustic window available and cause our scan plane to pass through the region of abnormality. Much of the time the Force was with us. We made many correct diagnoses and provided lots of useful information to referring clinicians and patients. But we also missed things and, to make matters worse, did not realize what we were missing. Since 1978, when we began using real-time scanners routinely, we have changed our thoughts about scanning and the way in which we conduct scans. We have abandoned the picture-oriented scanning process and have evolved a different approach to ultrasound scanning—the organ-oriented examination.

THE ORGAN-ORIENTED EXAMINATION

The concept of "organ-oriented" ultrasound examination is quite simple. As the sonographer performs the scan he or she concentrates on individual organs or anatomic areas rather than on external scanning coordinates. While scanning, attention is focused on an individual organ, and the scan plane is adjusted to get the most useful images of that organ. The individual organ is studied intensely during the course of the scanning, many images and scan angles are used, and a diagnostic impression is formulated *while the scan is being performed.* The images the sonographer chooses to photograph are selected to provide a record of individual organs rather than represent whole cross-sectional slices of anatomy. Relatively few pictures are made, and these pictures are obtained to illustrate the diagnosis rather than to record the examination comprehensively. Instead of being labeled with external coordinates, the photographs are identified by the organ or area illustrated ("upper pole, right kidney; common duct").

The organ-oriented examination is the logical way to investigate a patient. If we think about it, we are not really interested in slicing the patient up like hamsteak or a cadaver and then trying to put the pieces back together like some three-dimensional jigsaw puzzle. Rather, we are trying to examine the individual organs that make up the patient and to decide whether those organs are anatomically normal or are anatomically abnormal. Since each of the organs is located in a different position in the body and is best visualized by using different acoustic windows, it is only logical that a scan plane or section that produces a good view of the gallbladder will not necessarily make a good picture of the pancreas. Scanning orientations that demonstrate the common bile duct do a poor job for the right kidney. Most organs are not oriented so that they are best seen in the conventional transverse and longitudinal sections. Therefore it is illogical to attempt to study these organs by using a standardized set of scanning planes that are not particularly appropriate to any of them. It is easier, instead of trying to examine the entire abdomen in one process, to go about the examination in several small steps, each of which is custom-designed to look at a particular area of interest.

The organ-oriented ultrasound examination not only provides a better diagnostic study for the ultrasonologist, it also is much easier and more logical for the sonographer to perform. It is far simpler to concentrate on making good images of a single organ than to try to encompass four different organs on a single picture. It is easier to keep track of what has been done and what has yet to be studied.

Born again department: If you detect a certain religious fervor in all of this, you are right. We have been doing ultrasound scanning for 10 years and have experienced many dramatic changes and improvements in the decade. We thought the advent of gray scale was a truly momentous innovation that elevated ultrasound into the modern diagnostic imaging class. Since we have changed our scanning method to the organ-oriented approach we have seen a comparable improvement in our entire scanning and diagnostic process. In fact, we feel that the single most important thing an ultrasound laboratory can do to improve the value of its scanning is to use the organ-oriented scanning philosophy. Even if you are stuck with a vintage 1976 model scanner you will still improve your diagnoses.

ORGAN-ORIENTED SCANNING

Now that we understand the philosophy behind the organ-oriented ultrasound examination we can see that performing the scan is actually quite simple: There are five steps.

1. *Examine each organ individually.* An ultrasound examination is not a juggling performance. Just as it is difficult to keep more than one ball in the air at a time when juggling, it is difficult to do a good job of examining a patient when you are trying to look at more than one organ at a time. When scanning, your attention should be concentrated on one organ at a time.

2. *Examine each organ thoroughly and formulate a diagnostic impression.* To avoid sampling error you must sweep the scan plane completely through each organ, making adjustments in the acoustic window as necessary, so that no area remains unseen. It is often useful to use more than one scanning orientation or patient position to examine the organ. For example, the lower pole of the left kidney can frequently be seen well by using coronal sections that pass through the lateral abdominal wall just above the iliac crest; the upper pole of the left kidney, on the other hand, usually requires a scanning plane that passes obliquely through the spleen. The purpose of these maneuvers is to get a good look at all portions of the organ so that you can decide whether it is normal or whether it contains an anatomic abnormality.

3. *Document your diagnostic impression with one or more hard copy pictures.* The hard copy pictures of the examination should illustrate the diagnosis you have reached. Because of the thinness of the tomographic slice, it is not possible to make pictures that represent the entire organ. This presents no problem. All that are needed are a few representative pictures to illustrate the essential nature of the organ. This is analogous to taking snapshots to document a vacation. We do not have to have a movie of everything we did on the vacation; rather a few well-chosen snapshots can make a good record of the trip.

4. *When finished with the first organ proceed to another organ and repeat steps 1, 2, and 3: Continue in this manner until all the abdominal organs and any abnormal masses have been studied.* It is useful to develop some sort of general routine for proceeding through the abdominal examination. The exact order is unimportant as long as you are careful not to overlook any areas.

5. *Write your diagnostic impression of each organ on the examination worksheet.* This is a very important step in the examination process and must not be omitted. Remember that the hard copy pictures are selected to show highlights of individual organs and cannot stand alone as a complete record of the examination; some type of written notation is also required. We have found that a simple worksheet such as

is illustrated in Figure 5–10 works well. This sheet is filled out immediately following the examination and is kept, along with the hard copy pictures, as the "record" or "documentation" of the examination. It has room at the top for patient identification data and any tidbits of clinical information we may wish to record. The main body of the sheet lists the abdominal organs in sequence; following each organ is a box that can simply be checked off if the organ is normal. If the organ is not normal, there is a space to make a brief notation regarding the abnormalities observed. You should design a worksheet for each of the various examinations you perform. You may wish to provide more space for descriptions of certain organs or areas and perhaps allow room for a simple drawing illustrating what you have found. The exact format of the worksheet is not particularly important as long as it is organized to provide a brief, but complete, record of your findings during the examination.

As you can see, the organ-oriented scan is actually quite simple to perform. Because it proceeds logically from one organ to the next, it is easier to keep oneself oriented than when

ABDOMINAL/PELVIS ULTRASOUND EXAMINATION

NAME

ABDOMEN		Normal	Abnormal Findings
	AORTA		
	LIVER		
	GALLBLADDER		
	BILE DUCTS		
	PANCREAS		
	RIGHT RENAL		
	LEFT RENAL		
	SPLEEN		
	ADRENALS		
	LYMPH NODES		
	OTHER		

Figure 5–10. It is imperative to keep a written record of the ultrasound examination to augment the hard copy. We have worksheets for each type of examination we perform: This one is for the abdomen. See text for details.

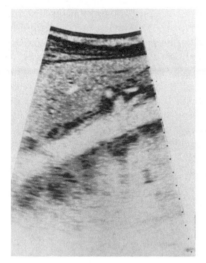

Figure 5–11. Upper abdominal aorta. See text for details.

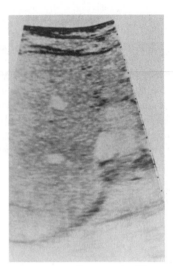

Figure 5–13. Central portion of liver. See text for details.

scanning in the more conventional manner. Just to be certain that we all have this procedure clear we shall run through a typical abdominal examination and see just what the sonographer does and why. The hard copy pictures of this examination are shown in Figures 5–11 through 5–22, and the worksheet is shown in Figure 5–23.

The sonographer begins by examining the aorta, starting near the diaphragm and working down to the bifurcation and iliac arteries. The aorta is normal, and a single longitudinal picture is made to illustrate this (Figure 5–11). Next, the

liver is examined, beginning with the left lobe and working toward the right lobe. Scans are performed in many different orientations and scanning planes, depending upon the portion of the liver being studied at the time. The sonographer feels the liver is normal and makes three representative pictures to show this; one through the left lobe (Figure 5–12), another in

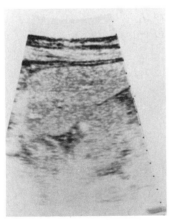

Figure 5–12. Left lobe of liver. See text for details.

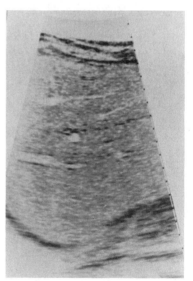

Figure 5–14. Right lobe of liver. See text for details.

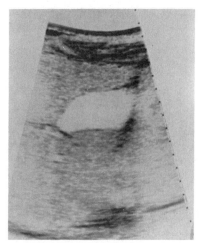

Figure 5–15. Gallbladder. See text for details.

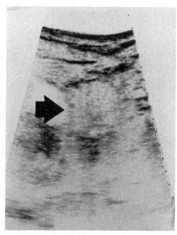

Figure 5–17. Enlarged head of pancreas in transverse section *(arrow)*. See text for details.

the central portion (Figure 5–13), and a third through the right lobe (Figure 5–14). The gallbladder is next. Rapidly panning the scanner back and forth through the gallbladder shows it is normal and contains no gallstones. Figure 5–15 is the single photograph taken. When finished with the gallbladder, the sonographer turns to the biliary ducts, which are traced from their intrahepatic branchings as far distally in the common bile duct as possible. A transverse section of the common bile duct just below its bifurcation is photographed (Figure 5–16). The

sonographer then looks at the pancreas and notices that it is larger than expected and is less echogenic than usual. Extra time is spent examining the pancreas in many sections, carefully searching for any evidence of a focal lesion or enlargement of the pancreatic duct. Figures 5–17 through 5–19 are the pictures made; each picture shows a different portion of the pancreas and demonstrates generalized enlargement and decreased echo production. The right kidney and surrounding retroperitoneum and adrenal areas are surveyed next. Here again, no abnor-

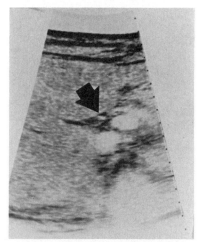

Figure 5–16. Common bile duct *(arrow)*. See text for details.

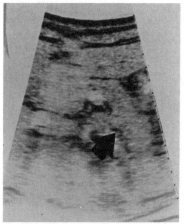

Figure 5–18. Enlarged tail of pancreas in transverse section *(arrow)*. See text for details.

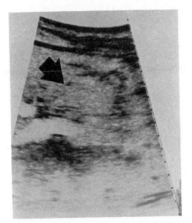

Figure 5–19. Enlarged head of pancreas in longitudinal section (*arrow*). See text for details.

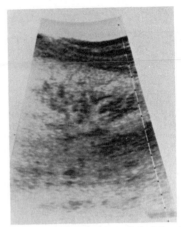

Figure 5–21. Left kidney with bifid pelvis. See text for details.

malities are seen, and Figure 5–20 records this. While examining the left kidney, the sonographer notices that there is a duplication of the collecting system, but no pathologic abnormalities. The hard copy picture of the left kidney (Figure 5–21) does not show the entire kidney but does display the bifid collecting system. Finally, the sonographer scans the splenic area and photographs it to show that the spleen is normal (Figure 5–22).

As soon as the scan is finished the sonographer takes the film cassettes to the darkroom for processing. While the films are going through the automatic processor, the worksheet is filled out as shown in Figure 5–23. Most of the organs are normal, and all that is required for these is a check mark. The common bile duct is measured and a note that its diameter is 3 mm is made. In addition to checking "normal" for the left kidney, an additional comment noting the bifid renal pelvis is made. The

abnormality of the pancreas is briefly described in the appropriate section of the form. By the time the films emerge from the processor the worksheet is completed and both the hard copy images and the worksheet are then taken to the ultrasonologist for presentation.

INTERPRETING THE EXAMINATION

By this time you are probably wondering if there is anything for the ultrasonologist (physician) to do. Who interprets the examination? Rest assured that the physician is still a key member of the diagnostic process. After assembling the pictures and worksheet, the sonographer brings them to the physician who will interpret the examination and presents the case. The presentation is brief but describes the way in which the scan was performed and the observations that were made and illustrated.

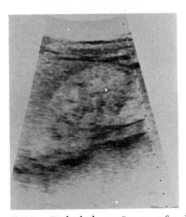

Figure 5–20. Right kidney. See text for details.

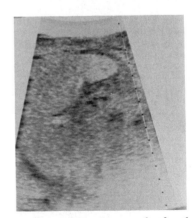

Figure 5–22. Spleen. See text for details.

ABDOMINAL/PELVIS ULTRASOUND EXAMINATION

NAME

WEBSTER, DANIEL   00-18-30
HANOVER, N.H.

ABDOMEN		Normal	Abnormal Findings
	AORTA	✓	
	LIVER	✓	
	GALLBLADDER	✓	
	BILE DUCTS	✓	(3 mm C.D.)
	PANCREAS		enlarged & edematous; duct OK
	RIGHT RENAL	✓	
	LEFT RENAL	✓	(bifid renal pelvis)
	SPLEEN	✓	
	ADRENALS	✓	
	LYMPH NODES	✓	
	OTHER		

Figure 5–23. A worksheet must be filled out for each examination. This sheet describes the study illustrated in Figures 5–11 through 5–22.

"This was a pretty easy patient to examine. The aorta, liver, bile ducts, and gallbladder were easy to see and all appeared normal. I am worried about the pancreas. As you can see in this picture and this picture, it seems to be too big, and I thought the echoes were less than those in the liver. I had a little trouble visualizing the head of the pancreas and had to come in from the side, but I think this picture shows it pretty well. I didn't see anything that looked like a dilated pancreatic duct or a mass or cyst. I thought the whole pancreas was enlarged, including the tail. The right kidney and adrenal region were normal. The left kidney is normal, but I thought it probably had a duplicated collecting system, so I made this picture to see if you agree. The spleen was a little difficult; I had to nearly roll him on his stomach and could only get a look through one set of ribs."

The physician listens to the presentations, looks at the images, and then makes one of three responses.

1. He* agrees with the sonographer's presentations, finds that the pictures are of good quality and believes they fairly represent what is going on, and decides that the patient probably has pancreatitis. He tells the sonographer to discharge the patient and signs his name at the bottom of the worksheet to indicate his acceptance. (Ideally he also immediately picks

*or she.

up a nearby dictaphone and dictates an ultra-sound report.)

2. The ultrasonologist agrees with most of the examination but is not certain about the pancreas. He decides to have a look at the area himself and returns with the sonographer to the examining room, where he repeats the study of the pancreas (and any other areas that are troubling). The rescanning usually does not take long because the basic groundwork has already been done by the sonographer, and the physician can concentrate on a few selected areas. The sonographer can also direct him quickly to the best scan planes for seeing problem spots. When the examination is finished the ultrasonologist may agree or disagree with the initial opinion of the sonographer. If he agrees, he congratulates the sonographer for the thoroughness of the examination, discharges the patient, signs the worksheet, and dictates the report. If he disagrees, he explains his reason to the sonographer, *changes the notations on the worksheet* before signing it, and then dictates the report.

"I think the pancreas is probably all right. It is a little chubby, but this is a young patient, and the pancreas can sometimes be a little prominent in people of this age. Also the clinical symptoms do not fit very well with pancreatitis, so I think we will just equivocate on this. I was concerned for a moment that we might be dealing with some enlarged lymph nodes, but I think you are right that the nodes are normal. That is a beautiful picture of the bifid renal pelvis, by the way."

3. The ultrasonologist decides to repeat the entire examination even though he basically agrees with everything the sonographer says. He does this periodically just to keep everybody on their toes.

Not all examinations are as straightforward as the one we have been using as an example. More often than not, there are areas of the abdomen or portions of organs that are not clearly seen, or the sonographer will be uncertain whether an organ is normal or abnormal. The sonographer will explain these problems in the presentation and ask the physician for help.

"This was a tough scan. The patient is fat and cannot hold his breath well. I could not get very good pictures of the liver, and I was worried that there might be an area of abnormal echoes here in the right lobe, but I could not see it well enough to be sure. Also the body and tail of the pancreas were a total wipeout."

"I want you to come back and have a look at this case. I keep seeing this echo in the gallbladder that I think is an artifact, but I cannot make it go away completely."

"This is an interesting case. He was just sent for a gallbladder scan, but when I was looking at the porta hepatis I saw these echo-free areas in it, so I checked the aorta and found similar echo-free areas there that extend along it. The patient also said he felt something in his left groin, so I looked and there are similar masses down there. It looks to me as if there are a lot of enlarged lymph nodes, but I want to have you check it to be sure."

In each of these situations the physician will go back and rescan the patient and work the problems out with the sonographer. As with the more straightforward cases, the physician can conduct the examination much more quickly because the sonographer has laid the groundwork.

Ad gloriam department: There is yet another physician response of which we are frequently guilty and which tries the patience of the most dedicated sonographer. "What a great case! I have been looking for an example of this for a long time. Get me some new film and set up the tape recorder; I want to make some pictures of this while the patient is supine, upright, swallowing water, and singing the National Anthem. Let us also put it on the videotape and record a bunch of discs for post-image processing, and so on. . . ."

There are, of course, an infinite variety of physician responses and interactions between physician and sonographer. The point to remember is that the sonographer does not act alone. The sonographer is an extension of the ultrasonologist and does most of the actual scanning procedure. Coming to a diagnostic conclusion and interpreting the scan is always the responsibility of the physician. In a good ultrasound laboratory the sonographers and the physician work together as a smoothly functioning team that can perform the scanning procedure in a rapid and efficient manner and arrive at an accurate diagnosis based on mutual observations.

PERSPECTIVE

Many physicians experience an initial malaise when presented with the concept of the organ-oriented scan. The distress will be especially pronounced in those instances when the ultrasonologist and his hard copies must compete with the lovely pictures produced by modern computed tomographs. In a conference where CT scans are the gold standard, the hard copies from the relatively limited field of view of real-time scanners will be at a disadvantage because they do not offer a global image. Always remember that we are seeking useful clinical information and that our product is not a pretty picture but a diagnosis. The information acquired in the scanning process is, therefore, at least as important as the hard copies.

Sometimes there is uneasiness about the role of the sonographer in the process and concern that too much responsibility is placed in the sonographer's hands. We often hear comments such as "I could not delegate that responsibility for diagnosis to anyone; I make all the diagnoses myself." At first presentation it may indeed seem that the sonographer is being assigned new responsibilities; this is not actually the case, however. The sonographer has always had a tremendous input in diagnosis by ultrasound scanning, regardless of the examination philosophy or technique utilized. The physician who feels that he alone makes the diagnosis because he looks at a series of pictures is probably deluding himself. While he may indeed be correctly interpreting what he sees on the images, he has no assurance whatever that the images were truly representative of the underlying pathologic condition, that they were performed with the proper acoustic windows and instrument settings to demonstrate small lesions, that important diagnostic information was not missed entirely during the scanning procedure, or that the pictures are not misleading owing to sampling error. The physician has always been placing tremendous responsibility in the hands of the sonographer by allowing him to select scanning planes, instrument settings, and which images to record. Just because the physician has eight normal images of the gallbladder on film is no assurance that a small gallstone was not missed because part of the gallbladder was not satisfactorily visualized.

The sonographer's responsibility is the same; what is changed is the acknowledgement of the vital role he or she plays in the diagnostic process. By acknowledging this role and placing it "up front" we have found that the sonographer and ultrasonologist work more efficiently as a team and that the sonographers themselves approach their work with an enthusiasm and diligence that reap large dividends for all concerned. The great advantage of the organ-oriented scanning philosophy coupled with real-time instrumentation is that the entire scanning and diagnostic process is much easier. Both the ultrasonologist and the sonographer will find that it is a technically manageable and satisfying experience to conduct an ultrasound scan. What formerly was a sometimes tedious and often confusing process of piecing together a three-dimensional jigsaw puzzle has been turned into a fascinating search for disease.

BIBLIOGRAPHY

There are many short texts on scanning techniques available, including the first edition of this one. They all use the picture-oriented scanning philosophy and hence are not useful for modern scanning. Other portions of these texts are valuable, but steer clear of any recommendations for picture-oriented scans.

Chapter 6

BASIC ULTRASOUND ANATOMY

Anatomy may be in close competition with physics as the least favorite ultrasound topic. Perhaps this is because the old idea of anatomy for anatomy's sake conjures up ghoulish images of the anatomist's dissecting lab with all its attendant unpleasantries. We have found that anatomy for the purpose of conducting an ultrasound examination is usually not a painful or boring experience. In fact, because anatomy is the basic tool with which the ultrasonographer works and the newer techniques of scanning make it easier to comprehend, the study of anatomy has had a kind of rebirth. Ultrasound images are, after all, only pictures of internal anatomy; and the purpose of the ultrasound examination is to detect alterations in this anatomy that announce the presence of underlying disease. Anatomy for its own sake may not be so interesting; anatomy for medical diagnosis is fascinating.

In order to recognize an abnormality, one must first be familiar with the normal appearance of the abdominal contents. In later chapters we will take up the specifics of individual organ anatomy and its appearance on the ultrasound scan, but before we discuss the details of individual organs, we must know how they are arranged relative to each other in the body and where to go about looking for them. This chapter reviews the basic orientation of the abdomen and pelvis with particular reference to those valuable sign posts, the major vessels. We will avoid excessive detail, but we must have some familiarity with major landmarks that are easy to understand. After all, one must know the ballfield before he can play in the game.

GENERAL ABDOMINAL ORGANIZATION

We shall consider the abdomen as that area that extends from the diaphragm down approx-

imately to the level of the iliac crests; the area from the iliac crests to the symphysis pubis represents the pelvis. The most common anatomic distinction made in the abdomen is that of **intraperitoneal** and **retroperitoneal**. While this designation is useful for the pure anatomist and valuable for understanding the pathophysiologic spread of some disease processes, it is not very helpful for ultrasound purposes. We find it somewhat confusing and prefer to think of the abdomen as being divided into a **ventral** ("toward the anterior abdominal wall" or "upper") half and a **dorsal** ("toward the spine" or "lower") half.

When-in-Rome department: The use of intraperitoneal and retroperitoneal anatomic divisions is widespread, and it is prudent for ultrasonographers, particularly those facing an examination, to have some understanding of these terms and which organs are located in which space. Very briefly, the peritoneum is a thin membrane that lines the belly, forming a completely closed space that has no communication with the outside *except via the fallopian tubes in women.* The peritoneum covers many abdominal organs, much as plastic wrap covers the hotdogs at your local supermarket. These organs—the liver, gallbladder, spleen, stomach and small intestines, transverse colon, uterus, fallopian tubes, and ovaries—are said to be "intraperitoneal" because they are more or less completely invested by peritoneum and project into the peritoneal space. The other abdominal organs—the kidneys, adrenals, pancreas, most of the duodenum, ascending and descending colon, urinary bladder, aorta, and lymph nodes—are termed "extra- or retro-peritoneal" because only one of their surfaces is covered by peritoneum and they lie outside the peritoneal cavity.

Figure 6–1 is a diagrammatic representation of the abdomen in transverse section. It is oval and is divided into right and left sides by the mass of the spinal column and the large muscles running beside it. The spine projects a goodly

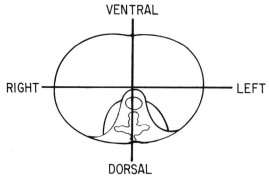

Figure 6–1. We like to divide the abdomen into four general regions: right and left ventral and right and left dorsal. Transverse sections such as this are always oriented as if we were looking up from the patient's feet; the patient's right side is on the left of the picture.

distance into the abdomen, much more than most people realize. At the level of the diaphragm the ventral surface of the spine is near the midplane of the abdomen, while down near the iliac crest the spine lies more than two thirds of the way to the anterior abdominal wall. If we draw a horizontal line through the level of the upper margin of the spine, we can divide the abdomen into ventral and dorsal halves. The anterior, or ventral, half is occupied predominantly by the stomach and bowel, most of the liver (the right lobe of the liver extends into the dorsal half of the abdomen), the bile ducts and the gallbladder, and the head and body of the pancreas. The posterior, or dorsal, half of the abdomen contains the kidneys, the adrenal glands, the tail of the pancreas, and the spleen. The aorta, the inferior vena cava, and the lymph nodes are located at the boundary between the two halves. In describing locations along the axis of the body we will use the term *craniad* to mean "toward the patient's head" and *caudad* to mean "toward the patient's feet."

In the anterior half of the abdomen the liver occupies the right and central portions, while the stomach occupies the left. In most people the left lobe of the liver is large enough to overlap a portion of the stomach, and when it does, it always goes anterior, or ventral, to the stomach—that is, the liver lies between the skin surface and the stomach. Similarly, the gallbladder lies underneath, or dorsal to, the liver. As we move toward the patient's feet (caudad), the ventral half of the abdomen is occupied by the small intestine and portions of the colon. Sometimes the gallbladder and the right lobe of the liver also project into this area.

In the dorsal half of the abdomen, the kidneys are symmetrically placed, although the left kidney usually lies slightly more toward the patient's head (craniad) than its right counterpart. On the left side the spleen lies craniad and lateral to the kidney; on the right side the same territory is occupied by the right lobe of the liver. The aorta and the inferior vena cava pass down the center of the abdomen, the aorta on the patient's left and the inferior vena cava on the right. They are flanked on either side by lymph nodes. The head of the pancreas lies in the ventral half of the abdomen just to the right of midline; the body of the pancreas crosses to the left and then dips into the dorsal half. The tail of the pancreas lies in close approximation to the spleen and upper pole of the left kidney. Figure 6–2 is a diagrammatic representation of these relationships.

The pelvis can also be divided roughly into

Figure 6–2. In the "typical" patient the organs of the upper abdomen all fit neatly together. This relationship of the organs is very constant; the only common variation is the size of the left lobe of the liver. Ao = Aorta, IVC = inferior vena cava, P = pancreas, L = liver, St = stomach, RK = right kidney, LK = left kidney, Sp = spleen.

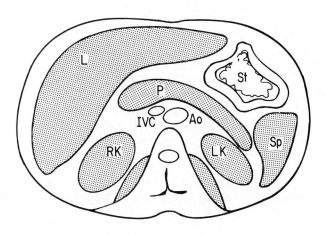

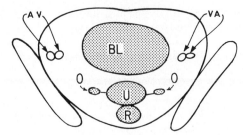

Figure 6–3. The ventral half of the pelvis is occupied by either the bladder or the small intestine. The former is an excellent acoustic window, but the latter is an acoustic wall. A = iliac artery, V = iliac vein, Bl = bladder, O = ovary, U = uterus, R = rectum.

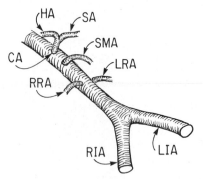

Figure 6–4. The aorta and its major branches are the most dorsal group of abdominal vessels. CA = celiac artery, HA = hepatic artery, SA = splenic artery, SMA = superior mesenteric artery, RRA and LRA = right and left renal arteries, RIA and LIA = right and left iliac arteries.

ventral and dorsal halves. The ventral half contains the small intestine, the sigmoid colon, the vessels and lymph nodes, and urinary bladder; while the dorsal half contains the female reproductive organs and rectum.

Applied anatomy department: Figure 6–3 is a diagrammatic representation of the pelvic organ arrangement. Looking at this figure we can understand why it is difficult to examine the pelvis unless the urinary bladder is distended. The ventral half of the pelvis is occupied by either small bowel or bladder. Small bowel invariably contains gas, which distorts and blocks the ultrasound beam; hence if the bowel is permitted to lie over the uterus and ovaries, it will be impossible to produce an ultrasound picture of them. In order to see these organs we must displace the small bowel by filling the urinary bladder, which will then provide an excellent acoustic window into the lower half of the pelvis.

ARTERIES

Discussions of ultrasonic anatomy invariably spend a great deal of time describing the major vessels of the abdomen. This is not because the vessels themselves are interesting or are subject to disease; rather, it is because the vessels are easy to identify and have constant relationships to the more important abdominal organs. The major vessels are, then, a road map of the abdomen, and sonographers must become familiar and comfortable with the vascular anatomy so that they can use the vessels as landmarks. This anatomy is not difficult if we think of it as being organized in three layers. Working our way up from dorsal to ventral (or from deep to superficial when the patient is in a supine

position), the vessels of the first layer are arteries.

Figure 6–4 is a diagrammatic representation of the major arteries of the abdomen. The main vessel, the aorta, runs just above the ventral surface of the spine slightly to the left of midline. It enters the abdomen through the diaphragm, passes beneath the left lobe of the liver, gives off four major branches, and then bifurcates into the left and right common iliac arteries, which continue through the pelvis and eventually pass out into the legs. The bifurcation of the aorta usually occurs near the level of the umbilicus (hence the disappearance of the aorta in the lower abdomen on midline scans). The aorta is quite easy to identify because of its location close to the midline, its thick walls, its echo-free interior, and its visible pulsations.

The first branch of the aorta is the celiac artery, which arises just caudad to the left lobe of the liver near the craniad border of the pancreas. The celiac artery is a short trunk that rises directly anteriorly and quickly splits into three branches. Only two of these, the hepatic artery and the splenic artery, are usually visible on ultrasound examinations; the third branch, the left gastric artery, is of no importance for ultrasound scanning and is usually too small to be easily seen. The two major branches of the celiac artery go in opposite directions, as illustrated in Figure 6–4. The branch that courses to the patient's right is called the hepatic artery; and, as the name implies, it supplies arterial blood to the liver and portions of the stomach, the duodenum, and the pancreas. The branch

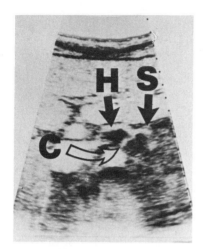

Figure 6–5. The celiac artery arises from the aorta and quickly divides into the hepatic and splenic arteries. H = hepatic artery, S = splenic artery, C = celiac artery.

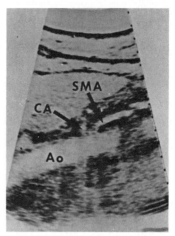

Figure 6–6. The superior mesenteric artery arises from the aorta just distal to the celiac; it runs parallel to the aorta and anterior to it. CA = celiac artery, SMA = superior mesenteric artery, Ao = aorta.

that goes to the patient's left is the splenic artery. The celiac artery and its branches have a typical T-shaped appearance on transverse scans, as seen in Figure 6–5.

The superior mesenteric artery arises from the aorta about 2 cm distal, or caudad, to the origin of the celiac artery. It initially courses directly anteriorly, but it soon turns caudad and runs parallel and anterior to the aorta within the peritoneal cavity. The superior mesenteric artery supplies blood to portions of the stomach, the pancreas, the small bowel, and portions of the colon. Figure 6–6 is a longitudinal scan through the aorta that shows the celiac and superior mesenteric arteries.

Biologic variation department: Congenital variations in the organization of the celiac and superior mesenteric arteries are frequently encountered. The most common variation that haunts the sonographer occurs when the hepatic artery or one of its major branches arises from the superior mesenteric artery, a so-called aberrant right hepatic artery.

The remaining branches of the aorta—the renal arteries—arise about 3 cm distal to the superior mesenteric artery and go laterally and somewhat dorsally to supply blood to the kidneys. They can almost always be identified on transverse scans, but are not as easy to see as the celiac and superior mesenteric arteries. Figure 6–7 is a transverse scan at the level of the renal arteries. Often a kidney will have more than one renal artery, and the origin of

these auxiliary vessels is not predictable; this variability in the number and position of renal arteries probably accounts for much of the difficulty encountered in visualizing them.

The aorta ends in a bifurcation that forms the right and left iliac arteries. These arteries course laterally along the sides of the pelvis to enter the patient's legs. Whether or not they can be seen ultrasonically is dependent upon the patient's size and the presence of bowel gas. If abnormally dilated, they will usually be visible; otherwise they are often elusive.

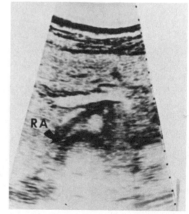

Figure 6–7. The renal arteries are often difficult to identify. They arise from the posterior-lateral aspect of the aorta and course dorsally toward the kidney. RA = right renal artery.

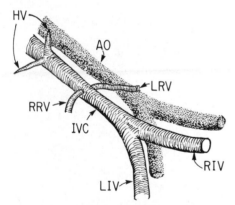

Figure 6–8. The systemic veins course parallel to the major arteries. IVC = inferior vena cava, AO = aorta, HV = hepatic veins, RRV and LRV = right and left renal veins, RIV and LIV = right and left iliac veins.

SYSTEMIC VEINS

The systemic veins returning blood from the legs lie in a plane just anterior or ventral to the arteries. Figure 6–8 is a diagrammatic representation of the systemic veins showing their relationship to the aorta. The inferior vena cava is the main channel and is formed by the junction of the right and left iliac veins at the same level as the bifurcation of the aorta. The vena cava then runs parallel to the aorta, anterior to the spine and slightly to the patient's right side. At the level of the kidneys the renal veins enter the inferior vena cava, and just before it passes through the diaphragm the hepatic veins join

it. Although it runs parallel to the aorta, the appearance of the inferior vena cava is quite different. It has thin walls, passes immediately dorsal to the substance of the liver, and is usually small when the patient is lying supine. The blood pressure in the vena cava is normally low, and this accounts for the collapsed appearance of this vessel under normal circumstances. The vena cava can be distended by having the patient hold his breath and bear down (the "Valsalva maneuver"). If the vena cava is distended or pulsates during normal respiration, it usually indicates right heart disease. Figure 6–9 shows the inferior vena cava in its normal state and following a Valsalva maneuver.

The renal veins are found at the same level as the renal arteries but are usually easier to visualize because they are slightly larger in diameter and have thinner walls. (This is a phenomenon that is observed throughout the body; when veins and arteries run side by side, it is almost always easier to visualize the vein than the artery.) Figure 6–10 is a transverse section through the renal veins. Notice that the inferior vena cava and renal veins are located ventral to the corresponding arteries and that the left renal vein passes anterior, or ventral, to the aorta.

The hepatic veins are the final tributaries of the vena cava and enter it just before it passes through the diaphragm. The hepatic veins are rather short and cone-shaped; transverse scans through the hepatic veins often have the appearance of the Playboy bunny with the head being the inferior vena cava and the ears the

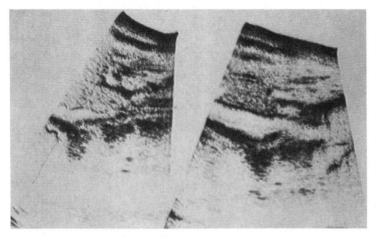

Figure 6–9. The size of the inferior vena cava can vary considerably, depending on the respiratory status of the patient: This scan was specially made to show this difference. The left half of the picture shows the IVC with the patient suspending respiration but *not* bearing down with the abdominal muscles; the IVC is not large. The right half of the picture is the same scan but the patient is bearing down (in medical jargon this is called a Valsalva maneuver), and the IVC is distended.

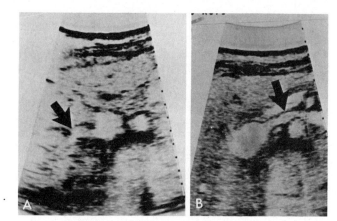

Figure 6–10. The renal veins are larger and easier to see than the renal arteries.

A. The right renal vein.

B. The left renal vein. Notice that the vein passes ventral to the aorta.

hepatic veins (Figure 6–11). The walls of the hepatic veins are not prominent; the veins appear almost as slits in the hepatic parenchyma.

The systemic veins receive blood from legs, back, kidneys, and liver. Blood that returns from bowel and spleen does not go directly into the systemic veins, but passes through the portal venous system.

PORTAL VENOUS SYSTEM

The portal venous system is the ultrasonographer's best friend. It is easy to visualize, has a characteristic appearance, and is the most valuable landmark for finding the pancreas and bile ducts.

The word *portal* means "passageway," and the portal venous system serves as a passageway for blood to pass from bowel and spleen into the liver. (No one knows why the body was designed so that blood that returns from the bowel passes through the liver before it returns to the heart. Probably the best explanation is that this blood is rich in nutrients from the bowel, and since the liver is the main processing station for body metabolism, it seems logical to give it first crack at any of the goodies.) The portal venous system is formed by confluence of the splenic and superior mesenteric veins, as illustrated in Figure 6–12. The superior mesenteric vein receives venous blood from stomach, small bowel, and colon; and its branches

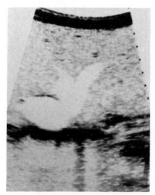

Figure 6–11. The short hepatic veins enter the vena cava just caudad to the diaphragm; on transverse sections they can look like the Playboy bunny.

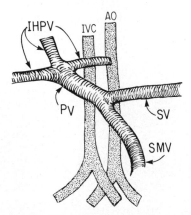

Figure 6–12. The portal venous system lies ventral to both the arteries and systemic veins. IHPV = intrahepatic portal veins, PV = portal vein, SV = splenic vein, SMV = superior mesenteric vein, IVC = inferior vena cava, AO = aorta.

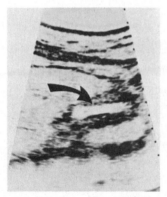

Figure 6–13. The superior mesenteric vein *(arrow)* runs parallel and ventral to the aorta and vena cava.

follow those of the superior mesenteric artery. The splenic vein receives venous blood from the spleen. These two vessels join together slightly anterior to the inferior vena cava to form the portal vein. The portal vein is rather short, usually only 3 to 6 cm in length, and passes immediately into the hilum of the liver via the hepatoduodenal ligament; here it divides into several intrahepatic branches. These intrahepatic portal veins distribute blood to all portions of the liver and account for about 80 per cent of the hepatic blood flow.

Figure 6–13 is a longitudinal scan showing the superior mesenteric vein as it runs parallel and ventral to the aorta. It is always larger in diameter than the superior mesenteric artery, and because its walls are thin it does not have

reverberation artifacts within its lumen. On transverse sections the splenic vein appears as a long tubular structure (Figure 6–14A). Like the superior mesenteric vein, it is a large, readily identifiable vessel with few internal reverberations and it is the *only large vessel in the abdomen that is oriented transversely.* (In a later chapter we will see how we use this vein to find the pancreas.) On longitudinal scans the splenic vein appears as a circle lying ventral to the aorta at the level of the celiac and superior mesenteric arteries (Figure 6–14B). The short portal vein is most easily found by first identifying either the splenic or superior mesenteric vein and tracing it toward the region of the hilum of the liver. In transverse scans the origin of the portal vein (that is, the junction of splenic and superior mesenteric veins) looks like a tadpole, the portal vein being the head and the splenic the tail of the tadpole. The portal vein is oriented at an oblique angle to the long axis of the spine, and in order to get either a longitudinal or transverse scan of it the plane of section must be altered appropriately. For example, cross sections *of the portal vein* are best made with a scan plane oriented parallel to the right subcostal line (Figure 6–15).

Once the portal vein has reached the liver substance it quickly divides into multiple intrahepatic portal branches. These are the vessels that we see in the hilar region and scattered throughout the liver (Figure 6–16). Many ultrasonographers worry about distinguishing the portal from the hepatic veins in the liver. We do not know of any compelling clinical reason to worry about this, but the distinction is not difficult. The easiest way to keep them sorted out is to remember that the hepatic veins drain

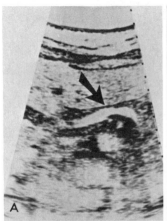
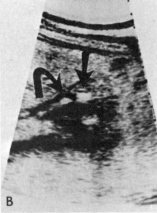

Figure 6–14. The splenic vein is the only large vessel that is oriented transversely.

A. On transverse scans the vein appears as a tubular structure.

B. In longitudinal scans it is cut in cross-section and appears round. Straight arrow = splenic vein, curved arrow = splenic artery.

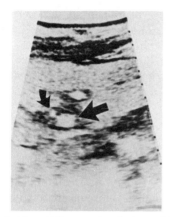

Figure 6–15. Oblique scans that roughly parallel the right costal margin will cut the portal vein in cross-section. Straight arrow = portal vein, curved arrow = bile duct.

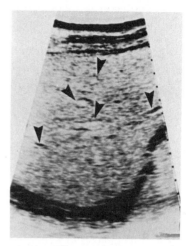

Figure 6–16. The intrahepatic portal veins are the small vascular structures we see scattered throughout the liver parenchyma (*arrowheads*).

toward the inferior vena cava near the diaphragm and hence will be oriented in an axis pointing in that direction. The portal veins, on the other hand, are oriented toward the hilum of the liver whence they arose. As we said earlier, the walls of the hepatic veins are thin, while the portal veins are thicker and more obvious. Portal veins are also more numerous than hepatic veins (when in doubt, call it a portal vein and you will be right most of the time).

THE PELVIS

Pelvic anatomy is straightforward but somewhat nonspecific. The main vessels in the pelvis are the iliac arteries and veins, and as we have seen, they are located laterally and define the side walls of the pelvis. In men the only visible pelvic organ is the prostate gland, and this can be identified only when the bladder is quite full. It is located at the inferior and caudal border of the bladder (Figure 6–17).

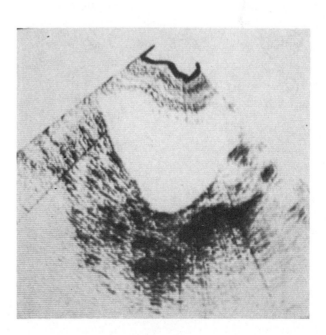

Figure 6–17. The normal prostate is located beneath the caudad, dorsal wall of the bladder. It is best seen on midline longitudinal scans through a full bladder.

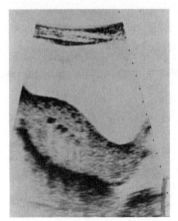

Figure 6–18. The uterus is located beneath the craniad, dorsal wall of the bladder. It is best seen on midline longitudinal scans through the full bladder. (The loud echoes in the middle of the uterus arise from an IUD.)

In women the uterus occupies the central area of the pelvis and lies immediately beneath the bladder (Figure 6–18). The ovaries lie to the right and left of the uterus, but their position is variable; sometimes they are found near the top of the uterus, at other times they are behind, or dorsal, to the cervix. We shall look at the anatomy of the pelvis in greater detail in Chapter 12.

PERSPECTIVE

Everyone who does abdominal ultrasonography should become thoroughly familiar with the vascular anatomy of the abdomen. Again, it is not so much that the vessels are involved in pathologic processes; rather it is that the vessels allow us to locate and identify the intra-abdominal organs. Work to become so familiar with the vascular anatomy that you can recognize the vessels in any scan orientation; this ability to identify the vessels will prove invaluable in finding such organs as the pancreas and the bile ducts.

BIBLIOGRAPHY

Carlsen, E. N., and Filly, R. A.: Newer ultrasonic anatomy in the upper abdomen. (Parts I and II). *Journal of Clinical Ultrasound* 4:85 (1976).
(We don't like the word "newer"—the anatomy is thousands of years old—but these are two excellent papers illustrating vascular anatomy. Dr. Filly has also published many other anatomy papers.)

Lyons, E. A.: *A Color Atlas of Cross-Sectional Anatomy.* C. V. Mosby Co., St. Louis (1980).
(There are many "cross-sectional anatomy" atlases on the market. This is our favorite.)

Chapter 7

AORTA AND
LYMPH NODES

This and the remaining chapters of the book are "clinical"; that is, they deal with the actual ultrasound examination of specific organs and areas of the body and how the ultrasonographer-sonologist team can arrive at a useful clinical diagnosis. We recognize that our organization is somewhat different from the traditional text-book format, which lists various diseases and then offers a brief description of the ultrasonic findings that are likely to be encountered. We admit to having a personal bias against that scheme. It works well in reference texts for the advanced student, but we have always found it confusing for novices. In real life when we scan we are presented with an image that must be converted to diagnostic possibilities. Without an already well-developed concept of what diagnoses are possible, it is difficult to use a textbook that is organized by diseases. On the other hand, if the disease process has already been recognized, there is no need to look it up in a book. In an attempt to get around this dilemma, we have organized our clinical discussions from the viewpoint of the ultrasonic appearance; beginning with a picture, we will work backward toward the possible pathologic processes that could have produced it. We shall first consider the aorta, the iliac arteries, and the lymph nodes. Because the aorta and the lymph nodes lie in close approximation to each other, they are readily examined as one "organ" in the organ-oriented scan. Also, there are relatively few types of diseases that affect the vessels or the lymph nodes; and hence this is a simple area in which to begin our exploration of the abdomen.

Aorta

NORMAL APPEARANCE AND SCANNING TECHNIQUE

We recommend beginning the examination of the aorta longitudinally near the midline. We start scanning up near the xiphoid process so that the left lobe of the liver can be used as an acoustic window; by gently moving the scan plane from left to right, one can almost always easily see the aorta as it passes through the diaphragm dorsal to the left lobe. The aorta normally has thick, echogenic walls; and its lumen measures between 1 and 3 cm in diameter, depending upon the age and the size of the patient. The pulsations of the aortic wall are also easily appreciated, particularly in younger patients. As we get older and our aortas age, the walls become thicker and somewhat irregular, and the pulsations are less prominent. The lumen of the normal aorta may contain faint, low-level echoes that arise from internal reverberations within the thick walls of the vessel (Figure 7–1).

It is usually easiest to follow the aorta by continuing the longitudinal scan plane down toward the umbilicus. Once the scanner has moved caudad to the left lobe of the liver, shadows and reverberations from overlying bowel gas may block the sound and obscure the aorta. When this happens it may be helpful to move the scanner either to the right or left of midline and angle the scan plane back toward the center. By looking "around the gas," one may be able to bring the aorta and para-aortic space into view. (Here the flexibility of real-time scanning is particularly useful.)

At the level of the umbilicus the aorta bifurcates into its two main branches—the right and the left iliac arteries—which should be followed as they track diagonally down through the pelvis toward the legs. Here, even more than with the aorta, it will be necessary to try different entrance sites for the sound beam in order to find a satisfactory acoustic window.

If there is any suspicion of abnormality or any difficulty in seeing portions of the aorta with longitudinal sections, the problem can generally be worked out by repeating the entire scan using transverse sections. In fact most

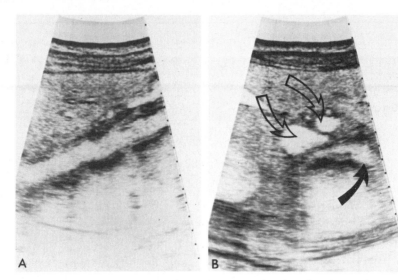

Figure 7–1. *A.* The aorta has thick walls and usually has faint "echoes" within its lumen. These "echoes" are actually reverberation artifacts arising from the thick walls.

B. Thin-walled veins do not have reverberation echoes in their lumens. The portal vein and inferior vena cava (*open arrows*) have "clear" lumens, while the thick walls of the aorta produce reverberation artifacts (*solid arrow*).

sonologists recommend routinely scanning the aorta transversely as well as longitudinally. The scanning motion is the same, a gentle side-to-side movement of the beam while slowly tracing the vessel from its passage through the diaphragm, past the bifurcation, into the iliacs, and out into the legs.

Loose talk department: It is one thing to talk glibly about visualizing the entire aorta and iliac arteries and quite another to do it. In many of our patients we are not able to see these vessels in their entirety, especially the iliacs, because of shadowing from bowel gas. Still, we can usually get a pretty good idea of what is going on and see enough of the structures to be comfortable in calling them normal or abnormal; fortunately, the most common pathologic process—aneurysm—enlarges the vessel, pushes the bowel gas aside, and is, therefore, easy to identify.

PATHOLOGIC APPEARANCE

Thick, Irregular Wall

In older patients the wall of the aorta is usually irregular and varies in thickness; elevated areas of the wall may project into the lumen, and some portions of the wall may be calcified and cast acoustic shadows (Figure 7–2). This represents the vascular aging process

known as **atherosclerosis**. The severity of this process differs from individual to individual, of course, and the mere presence of atherosclerosis and the raised wall thickenings (known as "plaques") is not necessarily pathologic in patients over 50. Sometimes, however, the plaque formation becomes so extensive that it seriously compromises the lumen of the vessel and decreases blood flow to the legs. Although disease this severe theoretically could be visualized,

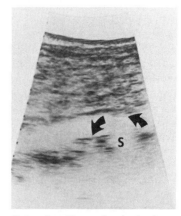

Figure 7–2. In older individuals the wall of the aorta is often thickened by atherosclerotic plaques (*arrows*). Plaque may contain calcium and cast an acoustic shadow (S).

there has not been much enthusiasm for using ultrasound scanning in simple atherosclerosis. The main difficulty is seeing the entire length of the vessel, because the acoustic windows in the lower abdomen are poor. As we have already explained, it is usually not possible to see all of the lower aorta and the iliac arteries, and consequently we often cannot fully evaluate the extent of atherosclerotic involvement.

Tortuosity of the vessel is a frequent accompaniment of atherosclerotic disease. In this situation, instead of pursuing its normal straight-line course, the aorta wanders to the left of the patient's spine, then back to the right. Unless one is wary, it is easy to mistake a tortuous aorta for a pathologic process such as a mass in the lymph nodes or an aneurysm (*vide infra*).

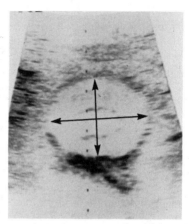

Figure 7–4. An aneurysm should be measured from outer wall to outer wall in both antero-posterior and transverse directions.

Focal Enlargement

By far the most common aortic abnormality is a localized enlargement or **aneurysm**. Aneurysms are really complications of atherosclerotic disease. As atherosclerosis weakens the aortic wall, there comes a point at which the vessel is no longer able to restrain the pressure of the contained blood, and it starts to enlarge like a balloon. For reasons that are not clearly understood this almost always occurs in the distal portion of the aorta, the area between the renal arteries and the bifurcation. Not uncommonly the aneurysm will continue past the bifurcation

into one or both iliac arteries; it is much less common for it to affect the aorta above the level of the renal arteries.

Figure 7–3 shows a typical fusiform aortic aneurysm. Frequently we see the remaining lumen of the vessel as well as the expanded wall. The echogenic area within the aneurysm is usually, but imprecisely, referred to as "clot." While much of this area is old blood clot, some of it represents bleeding within the wall of the aorta itself rather than a clot forming in a dilated lumen. These "clots" also contain many fibrous and scarred areas, as well as bits of atheroscleromatous plaque and calcifications.

The clinician needs to know three pieces of information about an aneurysm: its size, its extent, and whether it is enlarging.

To determine *size* the aneurysm should be measured on a transverse section at the point of its greatest dimension. When scanning it is important to remember to keep the scan plane absolutely perpendicular without angling it toward either the patient's head or feet; otherwise it will be impossible to compare measurements accurately. The measurement should be made from the outer echoes of the aortic walls and *not* from the margins of the residual lumen (Figure 7–4). Although it is easiest for the ultrasonographer to make the vertical measurement, it is also wise to attempt transverse measurement as well, inasmuch as this is what the surgeon is most familiar with and what he assesses when he evaluates the patient by physical examination. In most cases these dimensions will be nearly the same because the majority of aneurysms are round.

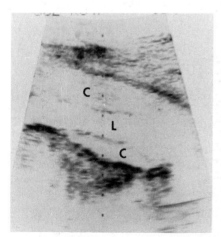

Figure 7–3. Aortic aneurysms usually have a normal caliber residual lumen (L) and an echogenic "clot" (C) composed of atheromatous plaque, old hemorrhage, and fibrous tissue.

Theoretically, it should be easy to determine the *extent* of the aneurysm. In practice, however, it is often frustratingly difficult to identify precisely the level of the renal arteries in patients with aneurysms. Knowing the location of these vessels is of considerable importance to the surgeon contemplating an operation because it is much more difficult to resect an aneurysm that involves the renal arteries than one that arises below the level of these vessels. For this reason it behooves the sonographer to try to establish the relationship between the renal arteries and the aneurysm as precisely as possible. Careful scanning in transverse sections is the most useful procedure here. If, despite your most diligent search, you cannot identify the renal vessels, try measuring the distance from the superior mesenteric artery to the craniad extent of the aneurysm. If this is greater than 3 or 4 cm, it can be safely assumed that the renal arteries are spared, because they originate close to the superior mesenteric artery. If it is not possible to determine the extent of an aneurysm accurately one must be honest with the referring clinician. It is far better for the patient to have an arteriogram to obtain this information than to have the surgeon be unprepared for the complexity of a repair operation.

Aneurysms that are not surgically removed are usually followed with serial ultrasound examinations to see whether they are *enlarging*. If there is evidence that the aneurysm is getting larger, corrective surgery is almost always recommended. For this reason reproducibility of technique is very important. We will discuss this in a moment.

What is the normal or "safe" size for an aneurysm? The most commonly cited figure is 5 cm. Surgeons have traditionally felt that aneurysms over 5 cm are at a high risk for rupture, whereas those below 5 cm are reasonably safe. Most of these measurements are made on x-ray films, however; and because of the magnification inherent in the measurement of the aorta on these films, it is probably wisest to consider 4 to 4.5 cm as the upper limit of "safe" when ultrasonic measurements are used.

What is the lower limit of aneurysm size? How can one distinguish a large aorta from a small aneurysm? Commonly, the abdominal aorta measures as much as 3 cm in diameter in older patients, and hence anything above this figure is usually considered to be an aneurysm. It is important, however, to analyze the contour of the vessel as well as the actual measurement. Some patients have large, ectatic aortas that measure 3 or 3.5 cm throughout their entire length but have no focal dilatation. These aortas do not actually have an aneurysm. On the other side of the coin, there are some patients in whom the aorta is no larger than 1.5 cm but contains a focal dilatation, usually in the lower abdomen; this enlargment is clearly an aneurysm. We feel that any focal enlargement, regardless of its size, should be considered an aneurysm and should be followed with serial ultrasound examinations.

How do you insure that measurements made today can be compared with ones made six months ago? We find it helpful to make hard copies that incorporate points of reference as much as possible. On longitudinal scans include the upper aorta leading into the aneurysm, for example. On transverse scans include a portion of the kidney if possible. Before beginning an examination, carefully review previous ones, noting contours and pattern of the clot, so that the new scans can be made to correspond to previous ones. It is important to note subtle changes in contour, because these are often tip-offs that the aneurysm is enlarging, even though its maximum diameter has not changed. Finally, before reporting the current scan, remeasure the earlier ones because the area of change may have occurred at a site other than at the greatest dimension. Rather than report only numbers, give in the narrative of the report an assessment of change (or the lack of it). Everybody loves a nice, neat number; but slavish adherence to the measurements alone might do the patient a great disservice. A change in the extent or the contour of the aneurysm may not be as frightening as an enlarging diameter, but it is just as important to the referring physician.

Paravascular Masses

Some aortic aneurysms slowly leak blood into the para-aortic tissues or may even undergo active and rapid enlargement (**dissecting aneurysm**). We are often requested to examine a patient with acute pain to evaluate the possibility of dissection. Unfortunately, we do not know of any characteristic ultrasound appearance that enables one to identify this process. The wall of the aorta is always widened and disrupted by an aneurysm, and it is not possible to say whether this disruption occurred suddenly or is chronic. Unless there is a previous scan for comparison, it is difficult to recognize when an aneurysm is in the process of acute dilation. If there is a mass adjacent to the aorta or iliac vessels in the region of an aneurysm, the possibility of leakage has to be raised. More often than not, however, these masses do not represent acute bleeding, but are the residual of a prior event.

A warning: One must be careful not to confuse a tortuous aorta with an aneurysm (Figure 7–5). This is less of a problem with real-time scanning because the scan plane can be moved easily so that the course of the vessel can be readily recognized. If the tortuosity is marked, the lumen of the aorta will appear to be widened, especially in the transverse plane. Remembering that the transverse and anteroposterior dimensions of aneurysms are almost always equal, whenever an *asymmetric* enlargement is seen you should check carefully to be certain that you are not dealing with a tortuous aorta.

Lymph Nodes

NORMAL APPEARANCE AND SCANNING TECHNIQUE

Below the diaphragm the aorta and the iliac arteries are accompanied by lymph nodes. The greatest number of nodes lie to the right and left of the vessels, with fewer nodes anterior and posterior. Normal lymph nodes are small and cannot be easily identified as separate from the para-aortic tissues. In normal patients, therefore, you will generally not be able to recognize them. When they are involved by disease, nodes frequently enlarge, and then they can be easily seen.

PATHOLOGIC APPEARANCE

Paravascular Masses

Almost invariably masses that arise adjacent to the aorta or its main branches are enlarged lymph nodes. In the United States there are two pathologic conditions that account for most lymphadenopathy: **lymphoma,** and **metastatic carcinoma.** (Infection, such as mononucleosis, can also enlarge the nodes, but it is a much less common cause.)

We have found that masses located predominantly to the sides of the vessels are usually lymphoma.

Definitions department: We use the term *lymphoma* to indicate any of the primary tumors of the lymph nodes such as Hodgkin's disease, histiocytic lymphoma, lymphocytic lymphoma, and the like.

It is not clear why lymphadenopathy in this disease tends to straddle the aorta rather than surround it, but it is probably related to the fact that there are normally fewer nodes on the anterior and posterior surfaces of the aorta. Lymphoma produces sonolucent lesions that can be easily mistaken for cysts. For this reason, whenever we encounter relatively echo-free or cystic-appearing lesions anywhere in the body, we place lymphoma high in our differential diagnosis. In fact, the presence of sonolucent

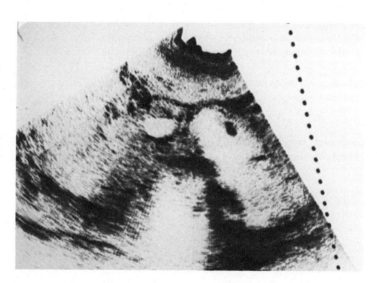

Figure 7–5. A tortuous aorta can be mistaken for a dissecting aneurysm unless careful scans are made in both longitudinal and transverse sections.

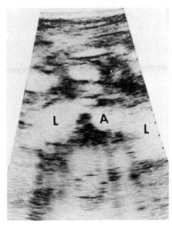

Figure 7–6. Para aortic lymphoma (L) often appears as echo-free masses. A = aorta.

masses situated to the right and left of the aorta is almost pathognomonic for this disease (Figure 7–6).

Circumferential Paravascular Masses

When a paravascular mass completely surrounds the aorta, creating a "doughnut" appearance, we have found that it is more likely to be lymph node metastasis from a distant carcinoma than lymphoma (Figure 7–7). Metastases usually have higher-level internal echoes and are less likely to appear to be cystic. Virtually any cancer can metastasize to the para-aortic and iliac lymph nodes, but tumors arising from the genitourinary tract seem to be the most common offenders.

There are some other uncommon conditions that should be included in the complete differential diagnosis of paravascular or circumvascular masses. These include **primary sarcomas of the retroperitoneum, retroperitoneal hematomas** (or hematomas from pelvic fractures if the masses are adjacent to the iliac arteries), **retroperitoneal abscess, retroperitoneal fibrosis, and hypertrophy of the psoas muscles.** Most of these can be recognized from their

characteristic clinical presentation. Hypertrophy of the psoas muscles is the only condition that occurs with any frequency; these patients are muscular generally have few or no symptoms, and the masses are bilaterally symmetrical.

PERSPECTIVE

Our observations on lymph nodes and paravascular masses are intended to be used as guidelines rather than hard and fast rules. While it is true that lymphoma *frequently* appears as paravascular sonolucent masses, there are many exceptions. Hodgkin's disease can produce an echogenic doughnut. Similarly a metastasis from lung cancer can be a nearly echo-free, noncircumferential, para-aortic mass. Whenever a paravascular mass is encountered the sonologist should give a *differential* diagnosis. He may then speculate as to the *most likely specific* diagnosis based on the clinical setting and the ultrasonic observations we have described.

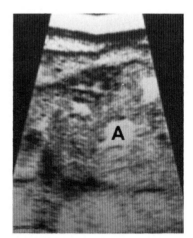

Figure 7–7. Metastatic tumor in the retroperitoneal lymph nodes may surround the aorta (and other great vessels), producing a "doughnut" appearance in transverse section. This patient had metastatic testicular carcinoma. A = aorta.

BIBLIOGRAPHY

Anderson, J. C., Balfoxe, H. A., and Wolf, G. L.: Inability to show clot: one limitation of ultrasonography of the abdominal aorta. *Radiology* 132:693 (1979).
(This paper discusses the problems that arise in using ultrasound to evaluate occlusive atherosclerotic disease.)

Wolson, A. H., Kaupp, H. A., and McDonald, K.: Ultrasound of arterial graft surgery complications. *American Journal of Roentgenography* 133:869 (1979).
(Ultrasound is the best method of following the aortic grafts used to repair aneurysms. This paper tells you what to look for.)

Hillman, B. J., and Haber, K.: Echographic characteristics of malignant lymph nodes. *Journal of Clinical Ultrasound* 8:213 (1980).
(Further discussion of pathologic lymph nodes; this paper emphasizes that the signs for differentiating lymphoma from metastases are not infallible.)

Chapter 8

LIVER

The liver is the key to abdominal ultrasonography because it is large, superficially located, and readily accessible to the ultrasound transducer. Its mid-level echoes provide a ready reference for evaluating the texture of all other organs. Furthermore, the liver is the main acoustic window into the upper abdomen; through it we see many of the important epigastric structures. The liver itself is the easiest abdominal organ to scan. In fact, if you encounter a patient in whom this organ is difficult to see, beware; it is very likely that the rest of the abdomen will be hard to evaluate and the examination will probably end up a bust.

NORMAL APPEARANCE

Anatomy

Anatomists and surgeons divide the liver into two main sections—the left and the right lobes—which are further subdivided into segments based on the distribution of the major hepatic arteries and veins. Many ultrasound texts deal in great detail with nomenclature and location of these various segments; and if you are preparing to take an examination, it is probably wise to consult one of these references to be certain of their definitions. From a clinical standpoint, however, the liver anatomy can be simplified considerably.

To begin, the **left lobe of the liver** lies roughly to the left of the porta hepatis, which, of course, is the site where the portal vein, hepatic artery, and main bile duct enter the liver. This lobe is divided into medial and lateral segments by the fissure for the ligamentum teres, through which in fetal life the umbilical vein and ductus venosus ran and carried blood back to the fetus from the placenta. In adult life the umbilical vein is represented by a fibrous cord (the ligamentum teres) visible only as a small round highly echogenic spot within the parenchyma of the left lobe of the liver. Everything to the left of the fissure for the

ligamentum teres is in the lateral segment of the left lobe of the liver, while everything to the right is in the medial segment.

Pseudonym department: The medial segment of the left lobe of the liver is sometimes referred to as the "quadrate" lobe because of its roughly square shape. This term is unfortunate because it is easily confused with the "caudate" lobe of the liver, which we will discuss in a moment.

The **right lobe** is usually larger than the left and contains about two thirds of the hepatic tissue. Everything situated to the right of the porta hepatis is considered in the right lobe. The main vessels serving the right lobe—the right portal vein and right hepatic artery—are oriented horizontally and quickly divide into anterior (ventral) and posterior (dorsal) branches, which feed the anterior (ventral) and posterior (dorsal) segments of the right lobe. (The right *hepatic* vein forms the official dividing line between these segments.) The medial portion of the posterior segment of the right lobe of the liver extends toward the patient's midline underneath (dorsal to) the porta hepatis and left lobe. This portion of the liver is known as the "caudate" lobe. Figure 8–1 illustrates these normal anatomic points.

The liver is unique among the abdominal organs in that it has a dual blood supply. The arterial blood comes from the hepatic artery, which enters via the porta hepatis and sends branches to all the various segments. The hepatic artery, however, supplies only about 20 per cent of the liver's blood flow. The remaining 80 per cent comes from the portal vein and its branches. All of the venous blood leaving the liver drains into the inferior vena cava via the hepatic veins. These veins themselves are anatomically unusual because they do not run parallel to the vessels that bring the blood into the organ as is the case almost everywhere else in the body. The distinction between hepatic and portal veins is not hard. First, they run in different directions. The hepatic veins course

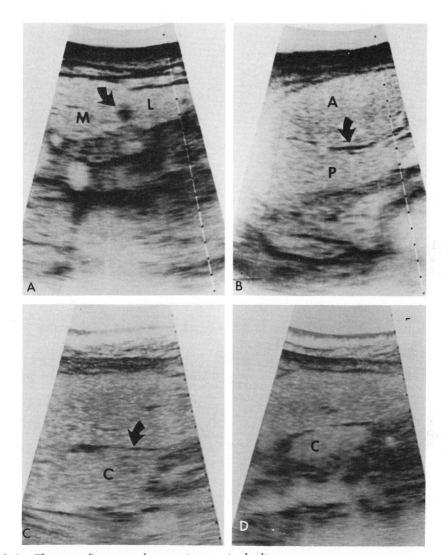

Figure 8–1. There are five general anatomic areas in the liver.

A. The fissure for the ligamentum teres (*arrow*) separates the medial (M) and lateral (L) segments of the left lobe, seen here in a transverse section.

B. The right portal vein and hepatic artery (*arrow*) separate the right lobe into anterior (A) and posterior (P) segments, seen here in transverse section.

C. The caudate lobe (C) is the posterior-medial portion of the right lobe and is separated from the left lobe by a fissure (*arrow*). On transverse sections such as this it is readily apparent.

D. On longitudinal scans the caudate lobe (C) can appear as a mass separate from the remainder of the liver.

toward the cephalic and dorsal part of the liver where they enter the inferior vena cava, while the portal vein branches are largest in the region of the porta hepatis and radiate out from there. Second, the walls of the hepatic veins are not well defined by echogenic margins. In fact, their walls are so subtle that the veins often look like simple echo-free slits or cracks in the liver parenchyma. The portal veins have highly echogenic outlines that reflect in part the fibrous tissue and fat that accompanies them.

Size and Shape

The size and the shape of the normal liver are variable. Overall, the organ is formed something like a pyramid with the apex pointing toward the right axilla and the base toward the left hip. Considerable variation in this shape is the rule rather than the exception. The left lobe seems to vary the most; sometimes it can be very prominent from the standpoint of both thickness and the area over which it extends, while in other cases it is almost nonexistent. It is, in fact, the size of the left lobe of the liver that most affects the quality of the ultrasound exam; a small left lobe will not offer an adequate acoustic window for seeing the pancreas and the left upper quadrant of the abdomen.

Texture

The liver parenchyma produces echoes of mid-level strength; normally its echogenicity is greater than that of the kidney, about the same as that of the spleen, and less than that of the pancreas. As we explained in Chapter 5, the sonographer should set the gain controls on the scanner so that the liver parenchyma is displayed as mid-level gray. Hepatic tissue is nearly homogeneous in appearance, and virtually all the echoes should be this same shade of gray. The liver, however, is not a completely homogeneous organ. Blood vessels and bile ducts run through it, and these structures with their highly echogenic walls and echo-free lumens are easily recognizable within the almost uniformly gray pattern produced by the liver cells. The resulting texture has been referred to as "inhomogeneously homogeneous" (Figure 8–2). This apparent self-contradiction is an attempt to describe the texture of the liver and serves to remind us that the echoes we see

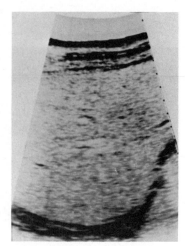

Figure 8–2. The texture of the liver is "inhomogeneously homogeneous": Small vessels and bile ducts interrupt the otherwise uniform texture of the liver cells.

come from different tissues. The echoes from the liver cells and their supporting elements are homogeneous, but they are interspersed with echoes from the vascular and biliary structures, which vary greatly in intensity (the liver is somewhat like a giant tapioca pudding).

SCANNING TECHNIQUE

We have found that in general the liver is best seen by scanning longitudinally; and we, therefore, always begin our examination with this orientation. We start with the left lobe of the liver and slowly work our way through the central portions over to the right lobe. The scanner is always kept moving, and we look at all parts of the liver—from the level of the diaphragm craniad to the free edge caudad. Representative hard copies are made, then the scanning plane is turned transversely and the organ is re-examined. Some ultrasonographers have found it advantageous to scan the liver in a plane more or less parallel to the right costal margin (the "subcostal" plane). This is made easier by turning the patient slightly up onto his left side. Regardless of the plane used, the trick is to make a thorough and complete search through the entire liver, stopping to record representative images, either to demonstrate that the liver is normal or to display areas of abnormality.

The upper portion of the liver is partially obscured by the overlying rib cage; therefore, the patient must take a deep breath to bring the liver down into the abdomen, out from under the shadows of the ribs. Unfortunately, this maneuver does not always work. The upper part of the right lobe of the liver may remain hidden underneath the rib cage, and the chance of missing something important is greatly increased. How does one deal with this? First, from either a transverse or subcostal plane the sound beam can be angled sharply craniad toward the diaphragm, and most of the organ will be seen. Second, real-time instruments make it useful (and possible) to scan up over the ribs. There has been something of a psychological barrier to doing this, probably because of the knowledge that the ribs are acoustic walls and often produce reverberation artifacts. The spaces between the ribs, however, provide good acoustic windows; and as long as the sound beam is passed through one of these areas, perfectly satisfactory images can be obtained. The resulting picture may appear as though viewed through a venetian blind; but, as we all know, it is possible to see things through such a blind as long as you concentrate on what is visible rather than what is hidden. By controlling the patient's respiration, the "hidden" parts of the liver can be brought into view, albeit not all on the same picture.

PATHOLOGIC APPEARANCE

Size and Shape

Because the normal liver varies so greatly, it is difficult to make any statement about abnormalities of size or shape. **Hepatomegaly**—enlargement of the liver—is probably one of the most abused diagnoses in ultrasound. Remember that it is the total *volume* of liver tissue and not the *area* of the liver in any single tomographic section that determines whether it is abnormal in size. We believe that to call the liver abnormally enlarged it must really be big—"four plus" big. Obviously, if the liver is everywhere (that is, if it flattens the right kidney or extends well over into the left flank to provide an unusually good acoustic window for the tail of the pancreas) we call it enlarged. Anything less tends to fall into the "normal" range. On the other side of the coin, there is just as much difficulty in identifying a small liver. More often than not, if you have difficulty seeing the liver, it is not because it is too small

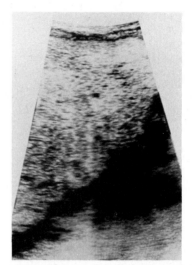

Figure 8–3. The margin of the liver should be smooth. When it is lumpy like this it usually indicates metastases. Notice the focal abnormalities in the liver texture; this is another good sign of metastases.

but rather because it is transversely oriented and hidden up under the rib cage.

Regardless of size, the liver's margin should be smooth and continuous. Any irregularities or "bumps" in the surface of the liver are likely to be pathologic. The most common cause of this type of abnormality is **metastases** as shown in Figure 8–3, but an irregular liver surface can also be seen in **cirrhosis**.

Texture

Fortunately for the ultrasonographer, almost everything that causes generalized hepatocellular disease in the liver increases echogenicity. **Hepatitis, metabolic disease, fatty infiltration**, and **cirrhosis** have a similar ultrasound appearance: They all produce increased echogenicity of the liver texture. (Some ultrasonologists have described decreased echoes in acute hepatitis, but this has not been our experience.) The best way to appreciate change in liver texture is to compare the echoes arising in the liver with those in the kidney and the pancreas. Remember that the normal liver has echogenicity slightly greater than that of the kidney and less than that of the pancreas. In the diffuse liver diseases just mentioned, the parenchymal echoes are increased and there is a striking disparity between the echogenicity of the liver and that of kidney. The liver may even be more echogenic than the pancreas in such cases.

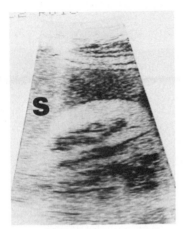

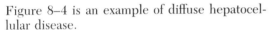

Figure 8–4. Hepatocellular disease causes the echogenicity of the liver to increase and become much greater than that of the kidney. Notice the acoustic shadow cast by the costal margin (**S**).

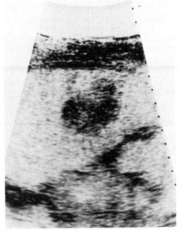

Figure 8–5. A benign hemangioma of the liver is a very echogenic, smoothly marginated lesion.

Figure 8–4 is an example of diffuse hepatocellular disease.

Because the increased echogenicity of the liver results in greater attenuation of sound, the beam often cannot penetrate as well to the deeper portions of the organ in patients with diffuse hepatocellular disease. This increased acoustic attenuation is another valuable clue to the presence of such a process.

We do not believe it is possible to distinguish among the various causes of hepatocellular disease on the basis of the ultrasound appearance, and thus we never give a specific diagnosis but rather a differential diagnosis in these situations.

Playing-the-odds department: The crafty ultrasonologist will make use of the fact that the most frequent cause of such abnormality in our world is alcoholic fatty infiltration and cirrhosis. Hepatitis and metabolic or storage diseases are much less common.

Solid Focal Lesions

Focal areas of either increased or decreased echo production in the liver are usually the result of cancer. The exception to this rule is the **benign hemangioma** of the liver, which appears as a quite characteristic single focus of very highly intense echoes with smooth margins (Figure 8–5). Hemangiomas are most often detected as an incidental finding on an examination performed for some other reason. All other focal lesions of the liver should be considered to be malignant until proved otherwise.

As you might expect, **metastases** may be either more or less echogenic than the surrounding liver. It has been said that hyperechoic metastases are more common than hypoechoic ones, but we believe that this may be a reflection of the fact that high-intensity lesions are more easily recognized. It is certainly true that many of the tumors that frequently metastasize to liver, such as those from the gastrointestinal tract, produce hyperechoic metastases. Nonetheless, many metastases in liver are echopoor rather than echo-intense, and the skillful ultrasonographer should be prepared for either type of lesion. Figure 8–6 shows examples of both types of liver metastases.

Identifying the obvious metastases is no problem; the trick is to pick up the subtle lesion. Unless you are aggressive about diagnosing metastases, you will have a 20 per cent false negative rate (that is, you will miss 20 per cent of the lesions). Remember that the normal liver is absolutely homogeneous (except for the vessels, of course); any heterogeneity in liver texture, no matter how subtle, should be considered suspect. We have found that maintaining a high level of suspicion has enabled us to improve our accuracy greatly in making this diagnosis. Figure 8–7 shows an example of subtle liver metastases.

Cystic Focal Lesions

Cystic or fluid-filled lesions of the liver are much less common than solid ones and may be due to simple **hepatic cysts, polycystic liver**

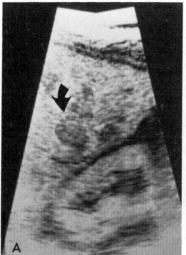
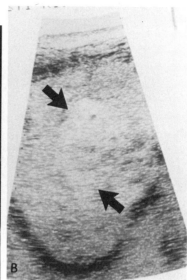

Figure 8–6. Focal abnormalities in the liver texture are nearly always due to metastases.
A. Metastases that are more echogenic than the liver.
B. Echo-poor metastases.

disease, hepatic abscesses, and **cystic or necrotic malignant tumors,** either metastatic or primary. Frequently the clinical setting and the appearance of the lesion will help you separate these possibilities. For example, polycystic liver disease may be associated with cysts in the kidneys.

As we have had the opportunity to look at more livers with ultrasound, it has become clear that there may be cysts in the liver that are not associated with disease elsewhere. It is important to be able to identify these lesions as benign and not clinically significant so as to avoid

unnecessary further invasive investigation. Simple hepatic cysts are usually isolated lesions with smooth walls and no internal echoes. They should fulfill the same criteria as a renal cyst as described in Chapter 11, if we are to classify them as benign (Figure 8–8).

Differentiation of liver abscesses from simple cysts or metastases may be difficult. Abscesses tend to have less fluid and more solid elements. Their walls are irregular, their margins are not as clearly delineated from the adjacent liver tissue, and through transmission of sound tends to be less than with simple cysts (Figure 8–9).

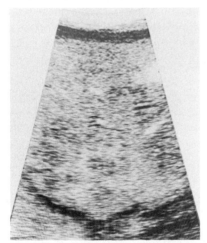

Figure 8–7. Any alterations in liver texture, regardless of how subtle, should be considered metastases.

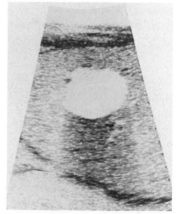

Figure 8–8. Simple liver cysts have echo-free interiors and smooth walls, and show increased through transmission of sound (acoustic enhancement).

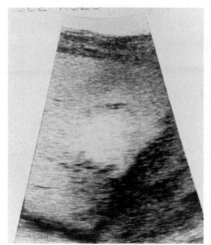

Figure 8–9. A liver abscess has irregular, poorly defined borders and some internal echoes.

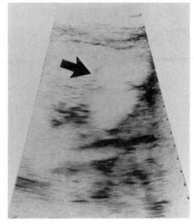

Figure 8–10. A necrotic liver tumor (*arrow*) may resemble a hepatic abscess or even a cyst. Fortunately this type of lesion is rare.

Also, of course, the clinical presentation will usually be of considerable help in making this diagnosis.

Tumors that are cystic or necrotic, like that shown in Figure 8–10, are uncommon; but unless the clinical setting clearly points to a benign lesion, we feel it is prudent always to consider this possibility whenever an echo-poor liver lesion is identified. If there is a question, it is usually an easy matter to perform a percutaneous biopsy for specific diagnosis.

PERSPECTIVE

As we have said, the liver is probably the easiest organ in the abdomen to scan. Once you have adjusted your eye to its normal texture or appearance, you should have no difficulty in recognizing the few things that go wrong with it. Just keep these three rules of thumb in mind: (1) Be wary of making definite statements about the size of the liver. It is only at the extremes of size that you can be certain that you are dealing with an abnormally large or small liver. (2) Learn to recognize diffuse increased echogenicity of the liver. Always compare the liver echo texture with that of the right kidney; and when the difference is quite noticeable, compare the echo texture with that of the pancreas. If the echoes of the liver are equal to or greater than those of the pancreas, there is diffuse liver disease. (3) Be aggressive in diagnosing liver metastases. If the liver texture is not perfectly homogeneous, suspect the presence of metastases until you have proved their absence by some other means.

BIBLIOGRAPHY

Marks, W. M., Filly, R. A., and Callen, P. W.: Ultrasonic anatomy of the liver: A review with new applications. *Journal of Clinical Ultrasound* 7:137 (1979).
(A complete review, with good illustrations, of ultrasonic liver anatomy. This contains everything you might want, even in your wildest anatomy frenzy.)

Gosink, B. B., Lemon, S. K., Scheible, W., et al.: Accuracy of ultrasonography in diagnosis of hepatocellular disease. *American Journal of Roentgenology* 133:19 (1979).
(A good discussion of the problems in trying to make a specific diagnosis of hepatocellular or generalized liver disease.)

Kurtz, A. B., Rubin, C. S., Cooper, H. S., et al.: Ultrasound findings in hepatitis. *Radiology 136*:717 (1980).
(These authors found a decrease in liver echo intensity during the acute phase of hepatitis.)

Newlin, N., Silver, T. M., Struck, K. J., et al.: Ultrasonic features of pyogenic liver abscess. *Radiology 139*:155 (1981).
(A good review of the appearance of liver abscesses.)

Chapter 9

THE BILIARY SYSTEM

The biliary system holds great fascination for ultrasonographers, both because it presents such a tempting target for the scan beam and because it is so frequently involved in disease processes. Here the emergence of gray-scale and real-time equipment has opened up the full potential for ultrasonic diagnosis and has established this modality as the primary means of evaluation.

NORMAL APPEARANCE

Anatomy

The biliary system collects the bile that is produced by liver cells and delivers it to the gastrointestinal tract. Bile contains two important types of substances: compounds that aid in the digestion of fat in the bowel and wastes that are being excreted from the body by the liver cells. Bile passes first into small intrahepatic biliary ducts. These intrahepatic bile ducts then join together to form progressively larger channels that eventually culminate in two main ducts—the **left and right hepatic ducts**—draining bile from the left and right lobes of the liver. Throughout their course the intrahepatic bile ducts run in association with the portal veins and hepatic arteries to make up the portal triads. (Although the channels run together, the flow of blood in the veins and arteries is into the liver, while the flow of bile is in the opposite direction out of the liver.) At the innermost part of the porta hepatis, the left and right hepatic ducts join to form the **common hepatic duct**, which then passes through the porta hepatis anterior to the portal vein and exits from the liver. Beyond the liver the portal vein courses toward the midline (to the confluence of the splenic and the inferior mesenteric veins), while the duct moves somewhat laterally and dorsally, passes through the head of the pancreas, and enters the midportion of the duodenum. About halfway along its course the

common hepatic duct is joined by the **cystic duct**, which leads to the gallbladder. The distal portion of the common hepatic duct, after it has been joined by the cystic duct, is known as the **common bile duct**. Figure 9–1 is a diagrammatic representation of the bile ducts.

Semantics department: While this terminology is useful for the anatomist, it is a bit pedantic for the general ultrasound examination. We prefer the term *main bile duct*, introduced by Weill. This refers to the portion of the duct that passes through the porta hepatis and includes both common hepatic and common bile ducts. From a practical point of view it makes little difference where the cystic duct enters, and there does not seem to be any money to be made by worrying about the true anatomic distinctions.

The gallbladder functions as a bile reservoir. During the periods between meals, bile (which is produced more or less continuously by the liver) flows into the gallbladder, where it is stored. When we eat, the gallbladder responds to the presence of food in the upper gastrointestinal tract and contracts to empty bile into the duodenum, where it can aid in the digestive process. The gallbladder itself lies just lateral and anterior to the main bile duct underneath the right lobe of the liver. In most patients the gallbladder is separate from the liver, but in rare cases it is completely surrounded by liver tissue and is then described as an "intrahepatic gallbladder."

Size and Texture

Most of the intrahepatic bile ducts are less than a millimeter in diameter and are thus below the resolution of abdominal scanners. The left and right hepatic ducts and their major branches can normally be as large as 2 mm in diameter and may be seen with the latest equipment. The lumen of the main bile duct averages 2 to 3 mm in diameter. Its size, however, is variable; and it is sometimes as large as 5 to 7

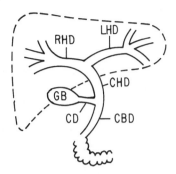

Figure 9–1. Bile, produced by the liver cells, flows into the intrahepatic biliary ducts, which converge to form the right and left hepatic ducts. The right and left hepatic ducts join to form the common hepatic duct, which runs out of the liver in the porta hepatis. It is soon joined by the cystic duct to form the common bile duct. RHD = right hepatic duct. LHD = left hepatic duct, CHD = common hepatic duct, CBD = common bile duct, GB = gallbladder, CD = cystic duct.

mm (more about this later). The cystic duct is usually small and short. Its diameter is never greater than 2 mm and it is difficult to visualize reliably.

The size of the normal gallbladder also varies markedly, as might be expected from what we know of its function. In a fasting patient the gallbladder can be as large as 3 to 5 cm in its anteroposterior dimension, but immediately following a meal it may contract down to almost nothing. (You can see that if one is to examine the gallbladder it must be filled; this means the patient should be fasting.)

The walls of both the bile ducts and the gallbladder produce high-intensity echoes. In the contracted state the wall of the gallbladder thickens somewhat and its echogenicity may decrease, although it still remains more echogenic than the adjacent liver.

The normal gallbladder wall is always smooth; any discontinuities or irregularities are abnormal. There is some controversy about its normal thickness, which we will discuss in a moment. For reasons that are not fully understood (including the effect of specular and non-specular reflections and variation in beam focusing), the posterior wall is usually defined more clearly than the anterior or side walls. Subtle differences in thickness and texture between the anterior and posterior walls of the gallbladder are normal. Many gallbladders have a partial septum that projects into the lumen, some are folded on themselves, and others have small valvelike folds near the infundibulum. All these common variations are easily recognized with experience, though at first they may be confusing (Figure 9–2).

The lumens of the gallbladder and the bile ducts are normally echo-free because they are filled with homogeneous liquid bile. Reverberation artifacts are, however, often projected into the upper portions of the gallbladder; these have a characteristic appearance in that they are always parallel to the anterior abdominal wall (Figure 9–3 and Chapter 4).

SCANNING TECHNIQUE

As we have already mentioned, it will be difficult to scan the gallbladder reliably if it is not filled with bile. To reiterate, this means that your patients will have to fast for at least six hours before you scan them. This can be accomplished by having the patient skip breakfast and performing the scan in the early morning (watch out for the cup of coffee with cream!). If the gallbladder is contracted, all may not be lost, but your job will be considerably more difficult. Examining the biliary system is an-

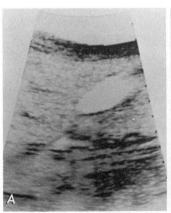
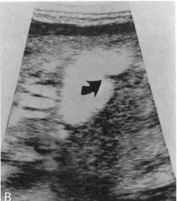

Figure 9–2. *A.* The normal gallbladder has an echo-free lumen and a smooth, continuous back wall.

B. The gallbladder may be folded on itself or have a prominent septation (*arrow*).

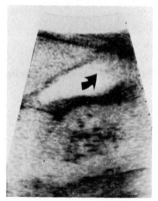

Figure 9–3. Reverberation artifacts from the abdominal wall (*arrow*) are often projected into the gallbladder.

other area where real-time scanners come into their element because of the ease with which the orientation of the scan plane can be varied. Following a small, elusive gallbladder or getting a good measurement of the bile duct is quick and easy. Also, because stones or polyps may be very small, the sonographer must be certain that all of the gallbladder has been visualized and avoid being lulled into a false sense of security by a single normal picture. The real-time scanner can be quickly swept back and forth across the gallbladder and ducts so that sampling errors will be less likely to occur.

We prefer to scan the gallbladder along its long axis and supplement the longitudinal views with cross-sections in selected cases. We always try to adjust the scan plane so that there is no shadowing from ribs or bowel gas. This is made possible in most situations by having the patient hold his breath in deep inspiration. Frequently, we will also have the patient roll up onto his left side because this moves the gallbladder out from under the costal margin more effectively.

Although many ultrasonographers recommend scanning the main bile duct in longitudinal section, we have found it easier and more reliable to scan the duct transversely. The structures in the porta hepatis—the main bile duct, the portal vein, and the hepatic artery—bear a fixed relationship to each other that makes them easy to recognize. In cross-section they look like the head of Mickey Mouse. Figure 9–4 shows this relationship of the duct, artery, and vein. The portal vein is Mickey Mouse's face, the main bile duct is his right ear, and the hepatic artery his left ear. Once you have this relationship in mind, it is no trick to find the duct quickly in nearly every patient.

It is best to begin by finding the portal vein (if you have trouble here, look for the splenic vein first, then trace it to the right and cephalad toward the liver). After the portal vein has been located, the scan plane should be rotated until the portal vein becomes as round as possible; the scan plane is now oriented for a cross-section of the porta hepatis. Usually you will recognize the Mickey Mouse figure immediately; but if it is not readily apparent, simply move the scan plane craniad—further up into the porta hepatis—and soon you will see the familiar ears. We like to follow Mickey as far into the liver as possible and make measurements of the main bile duct at the highest point. (Some sonographers in our department prefer to work backward. They begin by scanning high in the liver and follow the intrahepatic portal veins until they reach the porta hepatis and become the main portal vein. Then they rotate the scan plane to make the portal vein round and find Mickey's face.)

Once you have obtained the transverse view of the portal structures, you may also obtain longitudinal scans of the bile duct if you wish. This is done by placing the portal vein in the midportion of the field of the scanner and rotating the probe 90 degrees. You may be off a bit and will probably have to move the scan plane back and forth slightly until the duct is visible. You will recognize the duct readily

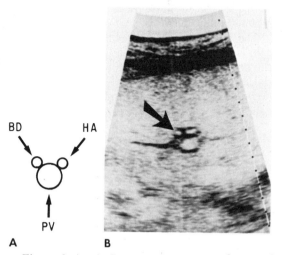

Figure 9–4. *A.* In transverse section the portal vein, hepatic artery, and main bile duct resemble Mickey Mouse. The bile duct is Mickey's right ear. BD = bile duct, HA = hepatic artery, PV = portal vein.

B. This transverse section shows a normal bile duct.

because it curves *dorsally* as it passes from above the portal vein through the head of the pancreas on its way to the duodenum. It is the only tubular structure in the upper abdomen that takes this direction; all the others shift *ventrally* as they course toward the feet. Any of you who have seen images of the bile duct on cholangiograms know that the duct is often curved as it moves from the porta hepatis toward the duodenum. Do not expect, then, that you will be able to see the whole length of the duct on one scan. (This is another reason why we prefer cross-sectional views for our initial evaluation of the main bile duct.)

PATHOLOGIC APPEARANCE OF THE GALLBLADDER

Size

The value of the size of the gallbladder as an indicator of disease has sparked controversy in the ultrasound world. While there are instances when size is an important clue to abnormality, it is not possible to set down figures that define a normal range for size. Once you begin to scan you will soon develop a feel for an "average" size and then will recognize when you are dealing with one extreme or other. On the upper end we feel that a diameter of more than 5 cm is *unusual*. (By "diameter" we mean the width of the gallbladder perpendicular to its long axis.) A gallbladder 5 cm wide or larger should suggest the possibility of obstruction in the biliary system.

Unfortunately, however, normal gallbladders may occasionally be that large, and an obstructed biliary system may be present without gallbladder dilatation. Thus a 5 cm gallbladder is only a "soft" sign of pathologic change. Small gallbladders are more difficult to define. Usually they are the result of some failure in the patient's preparation (the morning coffee with cream, for example), but occasionally one finds a shrunken gallbladder caused by adenomyomatosis, tumor, or cholecystitis. Fortunately, in these instances there are almost always stones and the wall of the gallbladder is usually thickened in a nonuniform way.

Intraluminal Echoes That Shadow

Figure 9–5 shows several intraluminal echoes that cast shadows in the underlying tissue. This is the classic presentation of **gallstones**. Al-

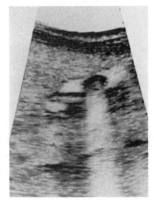

Figure 9–5. The "classic" gallstone produces loud intraluminal echoes and casts a prominent acoustic shadow.

though there are instances in which other pathologic processes such as **cholesterol polyps, carcinoma**, and **calcifications** in the wall can give this appearance, these lesions are rare compared with cholelithiasis. For all intents and purposes, therefore, intraluminal echoes that cast shadows are pathognomonic of gallstones. If the echoes and shadows shift when the patient's position is changed, the diagnosis is assured.

Some gallstones cast very prominent acoustic shadows, while others appear to have little or no shadow. Most ultrasonologists now believe that all gallstones cast shadows, but that it may be possible to demonstrate the shadow only if the stone is in the maximum focal zone of the transducer. In any event, we have found that stones that do not shadow are very uncommon and rarely pose a diagnostic problem. As long as the intraluminal echoes are mobile (as demonstrated by scans in various positions), the diagnosis of gallstones can be made with confidence regardless of the presence or absence of shadows.

Diffuse Intraluminal Echoes That Do Not Shadow

Figure 9–6 shows a gallbladder lumen with texture—faint, diffuse echoes that are located in the dependent portion of the gallbladder and do not cast shadows. We refer to this condition as "echogenic bile," although the term "sludge" is probably more frequently used. In our experience echogenic bile is usually *not* associated with gallbladder disease. (This is the reason for our aversion to the term "sludge," which connotes a pathologic process in most people's

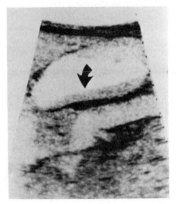

Figure 9–6. Echogenic bile (*arrow*) is not a pathologic condition. It is often seen in bedridden patients. (Notice the reverberation artifacts in the top of the gallbladder.)

minds.) Echogenic bile may be present on one examination and absent two days later. It is commonly seen in patients who have been fasting or bedridden, and recent work suggests that it is due to an increased amount of crystals (bile salt or cholesterol) in the bile.

Immovable Intraluminal Echoes

We believe that all gallstones should be movable when the patient's position is shifted. An intraluminal echo that is fixed to the gallbladder wall and does not change its position is either a **polyp** or a **carcinoma**, usually the former. All the polyps we have encountered have looked like polyps. They are either sessile or on a stalk, as shown in Figure 9–7, usually contain choles-

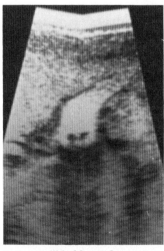

Figure 9–7. Gallbladder polyps are usually sessile but may have short stalks like the ones seen here.

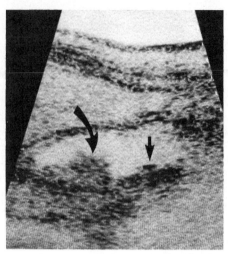

Figure 9–8. Carcinoma of the gallbladder is a large, fixed mass lesion (*curved arrow*) and is almost always accompanied by gallstones (*short arrow*).

terol, and are considered the anlage of gallstones.

Carcinoma of the gallbladder usually presents as a much larger, fixed, intraluminal mass that may invade and destroy the gallbladder wall and is almost always associated with gallstones (Figure 9–8). The lumen of the gallbladder may be completely obscured, and there may be evidence of growth of tumor into the liver.

Nonvisualized Gallbladder

Soon after we began to look at the gallbladder with ultrasound, it became clear that if the gallbladder were completely filled with stones, bile would be displaced and no lumen would be seen. Furthermore, the stones would cast a shadow, obscuring the back wall of the gallbladder; the only thing the sonographer could see would be a large acoustic shadow. We called this the "shadow sign" and found that not only was it a reliable indicator of gallstones but that it was the only evidence of gallstones in approximately 20 per cent of cases of cholelithiasis (Figure 9–9).

Other ultrasonographers have extended this concept and demonstrated that failure to visualize the gallbladder (assuming that it has not been removed), even if a "shadow sign" is not present, has a high rate of association with gallstones. Although we agree that failure to visualize the gallbladder is almost always due to cholelithiasis, there are those occasional patients who are very obese or who have high livers in whom the gallbladder may not be seen

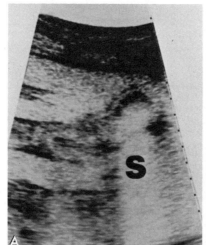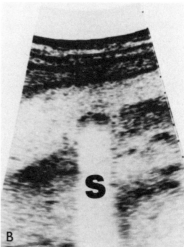

Figure 9–9. The "shadow sign" (S) is a reliable indication of gallstones.
  A. Longitudinal scan.
  B. Transverse scan.

for technical reasons. In cases in which the gallbladder lumen cannot be seen, therefore, we resist making the diagnosis of gallstones unless we are able to demonstrate the "shadow sign."

Thick Wall

The significance of the thickness of the gall-bladder wall remains controversial. Some authors claim that a thick wall indicates cholecystitis, while others have found no reliable association. In our own experience, the wall thickness is variable and measuring it can be fraught with problems.

In general it is true that when the gallbladder wall is inflamed with acute cholecystitis, it is thicker than when it is normal. The big problem is how thick is too thick? Three millimeters has been suggested as the upper limit of normal, but almost any patient in whom the gallbladder is contracted will have a wall this thick. Similarly, the gallbladder wall appears thicker in patients with ascites.

You pays your money and takes your choice department: The reasons for this are not clear. Some authors feel that it is because the ascitic fluid outlines the true outer margin of the wall; in the absence of fluid, the wall is underestimated. Others point out that the wall is thickened when the serum albumin level is low, a condition frequently associated with ascites. Still others have demonstrated that if the incident beam is not perpendicular to the surface of the gallbladder wall, the wall will appear spuriously to be thickened.

Because of these problems we hesitate to place much stock in the gallbladder wall thickness unless the thickening is localized, (in which

case **adenomyomatosis** or **carcinoma** has to be considered). Probably the best policy in regard to the gallbladder wall is to call it abnormal only when it is grossly thickened and contains some central lucencies or disruption. Obviously, if your patient has right upper quadrant pain, tenderness over his gallbladder, gallstones visualized by ultrasound, an elevated white cell count, *and* a thickened gallbladder wall, he has acute cholecystitis. If, on the other hand, your patient is old Bacchus, the village lush, who has cirrhosis, ascites, a low serum albumin level, *and* a thick gallbladder wall, his gallbladder is probably OK. The measurement of gallbladder wall thickness, like so many of the numbers bandied about in the ultrasound world, is no substitute for common sense and experience.

PATHOLOGIC APPEARANCE OF THE BILE DUCTS

Size

The main bile duct should be measured in transverse section at the highest level before its division into left and right hepatic ducts (Figure 9–10). If the duct is tortuous and that portion cannot be defined well, move distally until you get a good picture of the duct transversely and measure it there.

The normal size of the duct is controversial. (Is there anything in ultrasound that is not?) Some ultrasonologists use 4 mm as the upper limit of normal, while others permit a duct to be as large as 7 mm. We have found that 5 mm

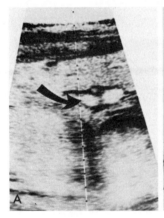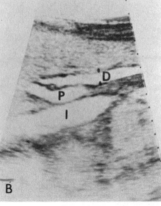

Figure 9–10. A. The main bile duct is most accurately measured on transverse scans. This duct (*arrow*) is nearly as large as the portal vein (Mickey Mouse's right ear is badly swollen).

B. Dilated ducts can also be seen on longitudinal scans. D = duct, P = portal vein, I = inferior vena cava.

provides a good differentiation between normal and dilated ducts. If the duct is 5 mm or less in size, it is not obstructed. On the other hand, when its diameter is more than 5 mm, the duct should be considered dilated *unless* the patient has had prior cholecystectomy. Patients who have had their gallbladders removed sometimes have a duct as large as 10 mm without evidence of obstruction. This does not mean that the duct enlarges after cholecystectomy; it has been clearly demonstrated that the main bile duct does not dilate after removal of the gallbladder. What probably happens is that the duct enlarged because of the passage of a stone and never returned to normal.

Main bile ducts dilate relatively quickly when obstruction develops, and one can expect to see them enlarge by 36 to 48 hours. The intrahepatic ducts do not respond as rapidly, and there may be great disparity between the size of the main bile duct and that of the hepatic ducts. Once dilated, a duct's return to normal caliber is much less predictable; it may never occur.

To summarize, then, we consider anything up to 5 mm to be normal for the diameter of the main bile duct unless the patient has had a cholecystectomy. In that case we accept a measurement as large as 10 mm. (We would make an exception in the postcholecystectomy patient if we saw the bile duct actually enlarging—going, say, from 5 to 8 mm between examinations.)

Obstructing Lesions

Figure 9–11 shows examples of the three common causes of bile duct obstruction: gall-stones, tumor, and benign stricture. The findings in each of these cases are fairly obvious.

A **common duct stone** usually causes obstruction at the point where the duct passes into the duodenum. When a duct is very dilated, the stone may appear as it does in the gallbladder, as an intraluminal echo that casts a shadow. Unfortunately, an obstructing gallstone is usually impacted in the end of the duct and is not easily identified. It is not that the stone is not in the image; rather, we cannot separate it from the adjacent bowel gas in the duodenum.

Tumor masses are usually easy to identify (unless they are very small) because the echo levels within them are different from normal pancreas. The longitudinal scan of the main bile duct is often helpful because it shows the dilated duct coursing caudad from the porta hepatis toward the mass in the region of the head of the pancreas.

Finally, **benign strictures** cause a smooth tapering of the distal end of the main duct with no tumor mass. When the end of the duct is clearly seen, this diagnosis can be made readily; but as in the case of the impacted gallstone, in a fairly large percentage of patients the distal-most end of the common duct is obscured by gas in the duodenum.

Although ultrasound is accurate in verifying the presence of obstructive jaundice, it is less valuable in determining the precise cause. If only all cases were as clear as those examples we have chosen to show you! Because of the problems already mentioned, however, we find that we are able to demonstrate the cause of jaundice in only 50 per cent of our patients. This has been the experience of most ultrasound laboratories.

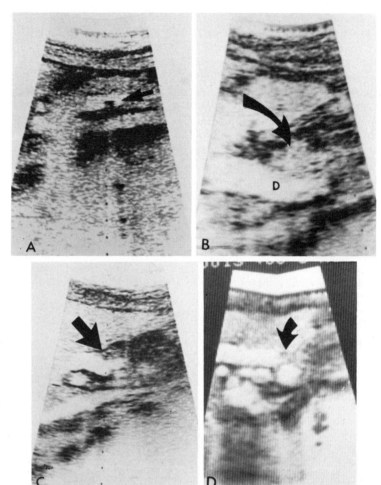

Figure 9–11. Obstruction of the bile ducts can be due to many causes.
  A. Gallstone.
  B. Pancreatic tumor. D-duct.
  C. Intrinsic tumor (cholangio-carcinoma).
  D. Benign stricture.

PERSPECTIVE

Because gallbladder disease is so prevalent, it will probably constitute a large part of your abdominal ultrasound practice. We believe, therefore, that it is important to provide some idea of the "state of the art" of ultrasound and the biliary tract.

Ultrasound is the best method for making the diagnosis of **gallstones**. Any ultrasound laboratory that cannot do a faster, more accurate job than oral cholecystography should turn in its transducers. The ultrasound examination is rapid and accurate, and does not involve radiation. The previous "gold standard"—the oral cholecystogram—has been shown to have a much higher false negative rate than was previously thought and is not as accurate as the ultrasonic cholecystogram.

Acute Cholecystitis (inflammation of the gallbladder) is a different diagnostic situation because well-established reliable ultrasound signs for acute cholecystitis are not at present available. Those authors who do recommend ultrasound scanning usually rely on the presence of gallstones and tenderness. Although it is true that the majority of patients with acute cholecystitis do have gallstones, the converse is not true. Most patients with gallstones *do not* have acute cholecystitis; and therefore, we think it is unwise to make this diagnosis simply because the patient has gallstones. Focal gallbladder tenderness is indeed a valuable sign in diagnosing acute inflammation, but you do not need an ultrasound machine to elicit tenderness; this can be done by physical examination. Other diagnostic findings such as wall thickness or sludge are not reliable signs of acute cholecystitis.

Chronic or **"acalculous" cholecystitis** is an even more difficult diagnosis. To begin, there is controversy among clinicians as to whether there is such a disease. There is no good evidence that the presence of inflammatory cells in the gallbladder wall causes symptoms in a patient, and there are no clinical studies that show that right upper quadrant pain in the absence of gallstones is improved by removing the gallbladder. Chronic cholecystitis appears to be a pathologic diagnosis, an incidental finding at cholecystectomy. The only suggested ultrasonic sign of this condition is a gallbladder wall of more than 3 mm thickness. We have already seen the problems with wall measurements, and this, coupled with the uncertainties about the existence of the disease, has caused us to take a very conservative approach. We never mention "chronic cholecystitis" in our reports.

Equal time department: We recognize that this is a controversial subject and that many people would disagree with our position. For this reason it is probably best for you to investigate the local bias and form your own opinion on the subject of the existence or nonexistence of chronic cholecystitis.

Differentiating **obstructive** from **nonobstructive jaundice** is very reliable with ultrasound, and this is now the method of choice for making the distinction. Unfortunately, ultrasound is not as good at determining the cause of duct obstruction, and frequently computed tomography or more invasive procedures such as percutaneous transhepatic cholangiography are required. We maintain, however, that ultrasound should be the first examination. In many patients the cause of obstruction will be demonstrated, and they can be spared further workup.

BIBLIOGRAPHY

Bartrum., R. J., Jr., Crow, H. C., and Foote, S. R.: Ultrasonic and radiographic cholecystography. *New England Journal of Medicine* 296:583 (1977).
(Our initial large, prospective study established that ultrasound was as accurate as oral cholecystography. Several subsequent studies not only have confirmed these results but also have shown the ultrasound examination to be more accurate than the radiographic one.)

Crade, M., Taylor, K. J. W., Rosenfield, A. T., et al.: Surgical and pathologic correlation of cholecystosonography and cholecystography. *American Journal of Roentgenology* 132:727 (1978).
(The Yale group showed that 96 per cent of ultrasonically nonvisualized gallbladders contained gallstones.)

Finberg, H. J., and Birnholz, J. C.: Ultrasound evaluation of the gallbladder wall. *Radiology* 133:693 (1979).
(There is lots of overlap between normal and diseased gallbladder wall thickness; it is hard to find a useful measurement.)

Goldstein, A., and Modrazo, B. L.: Slice-thickness artifacts in gray-scale ultrasound. *Journal of Clinical Ultrasound* 9:365 (1981).
(A discussion of an artifact that can cause the lumen of the gallbladder to appear echogenic. The artifact is caused by a poorly focused beam, and we have not found it a problem with our newest, well-focused scanner.)

Laing, F. C., Federle, M. P., Jeffrey, R. B., et al.: Ultrasonic evaluation of patients with acute right upper quadrant pain. *Radiology* 140:449 (1981).
(This is by far the best paper on ultrasound and acute cholecystitis. Unfortunately you must read the text carefully, since in the summary and conclusion the authors state that ultrasound is useful in making this diagnosis. Actually the study shows that the only valuable sign of acute cholecystitis is the presence of focal tenderness. Focal tenderness is a *physical* sign that does *not* require an ultrasound machine.)

Chapter 10

PANCREAS

Among ultrasonographers the pancreas is considered the test of champions. Before the advent of ultrasound there was no means of visualizing this organ in vivo; so being able to see the pancreas set ultrasonographers apart from everyone else. Now, however, computed tomography provides an alternative method of looking at this organ; and endoscopic pancreatography (endoscopic retrograde cholangiopancreatography, ERCP) gives an indirect look at the pancreas via the pancreatic duct. (ERCP, however, is a technical tour de force that requires considerable practice and expertise from the examiner as well as stoicism on the part of the patient.) Even though the pancreas is no longer its exclusive domain, ultrasound remains the primary modality for imaging this organ in the majority of patients. The pancreas is not easy to scan; but with practice, diligence, and a little ingenuity you will find that you can almost always do a very creditable job.

NORMAL APPEARANCE

Anatomy

The pancreas is oriented transversely with its head lying near the middle of the abdomen, just to the right of midline. The body and tail stretch out toward the left and pass somewhat dorsally and craniad so that the tip of the tail rests in the hilum of the spleen. The head of the pancreas lies directly anterior (ventral) to the inferior vena cava underneath (dorsal to) the liver (Figure 10–1). The head usually extends about 3 cm along the vena cava and is approximately 2 to 3 cm in thickness. Frequently the common bile duct can be seen passing through this part of the pancreas on its way to join the adjacent duodenum.

The body and tail of the pancreas have the same relationship to the splenic vein as the head does to the inferior vena cava—they run anterior (or ventral) to this vessel beneath the

left lobe of the liver or stomach. Figure 10–2 is a diagrammatic representation of the position of the body and tail of the pancreas relative to the splenic vein. This relationship is very constant; if you can make a transverse scan along the splenic vein, you will also be able to make a scan of the pancreas.

Size

The size of the "normal" pancreas varies over a wide range. In some cases the pancreas is flat and thin, never measuring more than a centimeter in any dimension, while in others it resembles a tadpole with a fat head and skinny tail. And in still others the gland has a thin head and body but a very bulbous tail.

In the past, measurements have been offered for the pancreas; usually 2.5 to 3 cm is said to be the upper limit of normal for any measurement of thickness in the anteroposterior dimension. We have never had much enthusiasm for

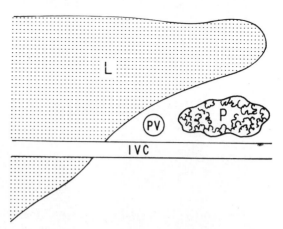

Figure 10–1. The head of the pancreas lies anterior to the inferior vena cava, posterior to the liver, and caudad to the portal venous system. IVC = inferior vena cava, P = pancreas, L = liver, PV = portal vein.

107

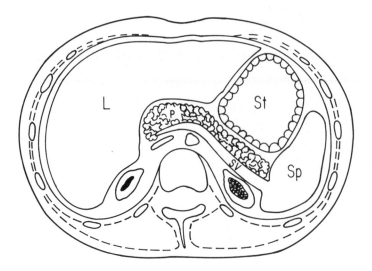

Figure 10–2. On transverse section the body and tail of the pancreas lie just above the splenic vein and underneath the left lobe of the liver and the stomach. L = liver, P = pancreas, St = stomach, Sp = spleen, SV = splenic vein.

such numbers because there is considerable overlap between normal and abnormal. While it is true that most pancreatic tumors or other abnormalities cause the gland to be larger than 3 cm in size, this is by no means universal. We prefer to examine the general echogenicity or texture of the organ and look for focal areas of enlargement or echo alteration rather than relying on an arbitrary measurement.

One step at a time department: We realize that it is difficult for the beginner to know what represents a focal enlargement and localized echo abnormality. With some experience you will have no difficulty in recognizing the great variety of normal shapes, and you will feel comfortable in separating the enlarged and normal glands. In the meantime, it is perfectly acceptable to use measurements as a temporary crutch while you gain experience. We suggest 2.5 cm as the upper limit of normal thickness for the body and tail of the pancreas and 3 cm for the head.

Texture

There is also considerable variability in the texture or echogenicity of the normal pancreas. In young people it commonly produces uniform echoes of moderate intensity that are only slightly louder than those produced by the liver parenchyma (Figure 10–3A). In older patients, however, the pancreas is more echogenic, and the intensity of the echoes becomes much greater than that of the liver; there may also be some mild heterogeneity to the echo pattern (Figure 10–3B).

Both the medium-intensity and the high-intensity echo textures are normal. The reason for the varying appearance is not completely understood, but most ultrasonologists believe that the texture of the pancreas reflects the amount of fat within its tissue. Figure 10–4 shows two CT scans of normal pancreas, one in

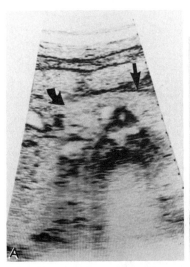
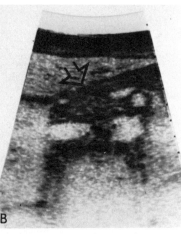

Figure 10–3. The echogenicity of the pancreas varies considerably.

A. A normal pancreas (transverse section) with low-level internal echoes. This texture is common in younger persons.

B. A normal pancreas with high-intensity internal echoes. This texture is more common in older individuals.

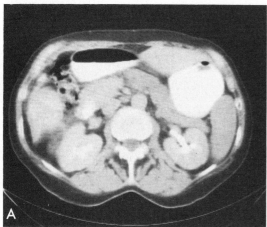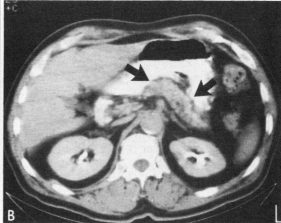

Figure 10–4. CT scans illustrate the probable reason for the variability in pancreatic texture.
A. The pancreas in a young patient is of uniform density.
B. The pancreas in another patient is infiltrated with ribbons of low-intensity fat. This tissue heterogeneity should produce high-intensity echoes.

a young patient, the other in an older individual. The young patient has a uniform, homogeneous gland composed entirely of pancreatic tissue, while the older subject's pancreas has been invaded by rivulets of fat, which seems to be a part of the normal aging process. Since fat is considerably less dense than pancreatic tissue, its presence within the organ gives rise to interfaces between tissues of greatly different acoustic impedance; and consequently, the pancreatic echoes are more intense. The exact mechanism of the variation is unimportant as long as you remember that the normal pancreatic texture covers a wide spectrum. We (and others) have observed that the *echogenicity of the normal pancreas is always equal to or greater than that of the adjacent liver.* If the echo intensity of the pancreas is greater than that of the liver, it should not be considered abnormal regardless of how great the difference.

Pancreatic Duct

There is controversy about whether it is possible to visualize the lumen of the normal pancreatic duct. We do not believe that the duct can usually be seen unless it is pathologically dilated. On several occasions we have conducted studies trying to identify the duct in the normal pancreas and have not been successful in the majority of patients. One can always pick two closely spaced echoes and say "aha! There is the lumen of the duct." Well, maybe it is and maybe it is not. We want to be certain that we are seeing the duct before we

call it, and therefore we feel that the duct must be visible over at least 2 to 3 cm of its length in transverse sections or must be seen as an entire circle in longitudinal sections. It is our view that when these stringent criteria are employed the lumen of the duct cannot be recognized unless it is abnormally dilated.

Even if the lumen is not visible, the area of the pancreatic duct can be seen in the majority of patients: It appears as a dense echo line running through the pancreas (Figure 10–5). Perhaps the whole controversy is really one of semantics. It is possible to see the area in which the pancreatic duct passes and, by inference, the walls of the duct itself; but it is not possible to see the lumen of the duct in the normal pancreas.

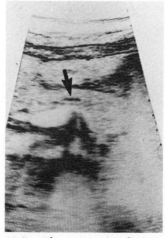

Figure 10–5. The pancreatic duct appears as a line running in the center of the pancreatic tissue (*arrow*) on transverse scans. The lumen is not seen in normal patients.

SCANNING TECHNIQUE

Technique is all-important in scanning the pancreas. Like the aorta, the pancreas is affected by relatively few pathologic conditions, and they are, by and large, easily differentiated once you have a picture of them. The whole trick in pancreatic ultrasonography is to get a good look at the organ. Because the pancreas does not have a capsule or other well-defined boundary and its texture is quite variable, it can be difficult to recognize with certainty. Fortunately, the constant anatomic relationship between the pancreas and its neighbors provides us with a sure-fire method of locating our target.

Recall that the head of the pancreas runs parallel to the inferior vena cava and just anterior to it. Longitudinal scans through the midportion of the liver, along the axis of the vena cava, will usually demonstrate the head of the pancreas (Figure 10–6). Sometimes air in the antrum of the stomach or the duodenum obscures the view, and it is then necessary to shift the entrance point of the scan to the right or left, seeking a better acoustic window. As long as your picture includes the inferior vena cava, you will almost always have the head of the pancreas as well.

Figure 10–7 shows the ideal way to scan the body and tail of the pancreas. The scan plane is oriented transversely so that the left lobe of the liver serves as an acoustic window and is adjusted so that the splenic vein is seen longitudinally. The echoes lying between the splenic vein and the undersurface of the liver represent

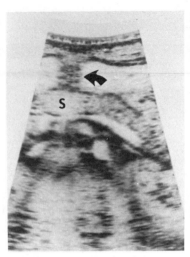

Figure 10–7. When the left lobe of the liver is large and the stomach does not contain air, the body and tail of the pancreas can be well seen on transverse scans. Notice the shadow (S) cast by the fissure for the ligamentum teres (*arrow*).

the pancreas. Once this scan plane has been located, the transducer can be moved back and forth so that all portions of the gland are examined. Unfortunately, scans like Figure 10–7 represent the ideal and are often impossible to produce. If the patient's liver has a large left lobe, the stomach and its air will be pushed aside, and there will be a good acoustic window into the left side of the abdomen. Unfortunately, this occurs in only about 10 per cent of patients. The other 90 per cent have smaller left lobes, and the stomach will cover varying portions of the tail or body of the pancreas. The stomach nearly always contains air that casts an acoustic shadow and blocks the view of the body and tail (Figure 10–8). If you are not completely clear as to why it is hard to scan the body and tail of the pancreas, look again at Figure 10–2, keeping in mind that the liver is an acoustic window and the stomach, which usually contains air, is an acoustic wall. It is important that you understand the cause of this problem thoroughly; otherwise you may be lost in the next few paragraphs.

We see that when a problem arises in scanning the body and tail of the pancreas it is almost always because of the absence of an effective acoustic window. Unless there is a large left lobe of the liver, we cannot see through to the tail. What can be done about this? Countless remedies have been proposed and championed over the years.

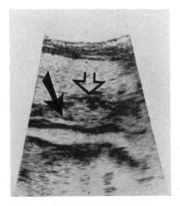

Figure 10–6. The head of the pancreas (*open arrow*) is best seen on longitudinal scans in the plane of the inferior vena cava. Notice the common bile duct running through the cranial-posterior portion of the head (*solid arrow*).

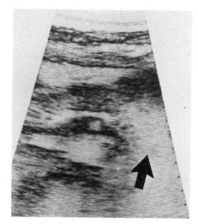

Figure 10–8. In most patients the tail of the pancreas is obscured by the shadow from air in the stomach (*arrow*). Transverse section.

The obvious approach is to give the patient several glasses of water or some other liquid to drink; after all, filling the stomach with fluid should turn it into a very nice acoustic window. Unfortunately, in our experience this procedure (which sounds so simple) does not work well. There are two problems. First, it is not easy for many patients to drink large amounts of water.

Do unto others department: If you do not believe this, try it for yourself. Go drink two 16 ounce glasses of water as is recommended in the literature. After you have returned from the bathroom, you can continue reading.

Second, while the patients are drinking water they are also swallowing some air, and as soon as they lie down, this air floats to the top of the stomach, providing just as effective an acoustic wall as ever. Having the stomach filled with water is of little value as long as there is air floating on top. Maybe we could move the offending air out of the way? If the patient were placed in a left posterior oblique postion, the air should rise to the antrum or duodenum, leaving only fluid over the tail of the pancreas. This is an attractive hypothesis, but it, too, does not work well in practice. By the time the patient is turned enough to get the air out of the way, he is usually so far over on his side that it is difficult to find a place to put the transducer. A further variation of this approach is to scan the patient in the upright position, which should allow the offending air to rise up near the diaphragm, leaving only fluid in the portion of the stomach overlying the tail of the

pancreas. We were so enthusiastic for this idea that in 1976 we had an upright scanning table built to accommodate patients. Even with this contraption we did not have much luck with our upright scanning. Either there was too much air to float completely out of the way, or the stomach, which is mobile, fell down into the central abdomen where it could no longer provide an acoustic window for the pancreas. Whatever the reason, our fancy upright scanning table has proved of little use to us and is just another of those items that stand around cluttering up the scanning room. Some authors recommend passing a nasogastric tube into the stomach to draw off the air. This method may work in some instances, but is not really practical for use in most busy ultrasound labs, and it is certainly unpleasant for the patients. Antifoaming agents such as simethicone have been suggested. These potions convert many small bubbles into one large bubble, but do not really address the problem of removing the air itself and have proved to be ineffective. Other investigators have suggested paralyzing the stomach with glucagon and then distending it with water. This method has all the disadvantages of simple water ingestion described earlier and, in addition, requires an intravenous injection.

Different strokes department: In 1973, in Denmark, we were experimenting with methods for converting the stomach to an acoustic window and tried, among other things, having the patient swallow a gastric balloon on the end of a catheter. The balloon was then filled with water through the catheter. Standard gastric balloons did not work very well, however, because they were too rigid to conform to the contour of the stomach and small pockets of air got trapped between the balloon and the wall of the stomach. In a temporary flash of brilliance someone suggested substituting a condom for the gastric balloon. Things went quite well at first; the flaccid walls of the condom conformed nicely to the stomach; and, when we filled it with a liter of water, we had a beautiful sonic window and could see the tail of the pancreas clearly. We ran into problems when we tried to remove the condom, however; no matter how much we aspirated on the filling tube we could not get the water out. There is no need to go into the terrifying details of what followed; suffice it to say that we were eventually able to remove the condom but have never tried this approach again.

As you can see there does not seem to be any good reliable method of converting the stomach into a useful acoustic window. If we are going to see the tail of the pancreas, we will have to find some other organ to serve as a port

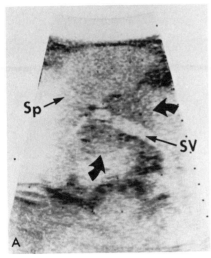
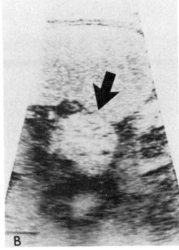

Figure 10–9. *A.* The tail of the pancreas (*arrows*) can sometimes be seen by scanning through the spleen. Sp = spleen, SV = splenic vein.

B. There is a carcinoma in the tail of this pancreas (*arrow*); the spleen is serving as the acoustic window.

of entry. Sometimes the spleen works well. By rolling the patient up on his right side and adjusting the position of the scan beam so it passes between the ribs and through the spleen at the level of the hilum, the tip of the tail of the pancreas can be seen tucked between the hilum of the spleen and the upper pole of the left kidney (Figure 10–9). As you will see in Chapter 11, however, the spleen itself is not always easy to visualize, and we frequently find that the spleen either is too small or is not positioned suitably to provide us with an acoustic window for the pancreas.

We have had the most success using the left lobe of the liver as our acoustic window and adjusting the scan plane so that it avoids the stomach. We call this approach the "down-the-tail" view of the pancreas. The concept is rather simple. The scans are all performed in longitudinal section. Figure 10–10 shows the liver, splenic vein, and pancreas in a longitudinal section near the midline. The pancreas is seen in cross-section and is reliably identified by finding the splenic vein and the undersurface of the liver. If the left lobe of the liver extended over to the patient's left side, we could simply slide the scanner from the midline over to the patient's left and follow the pancreas from the body through the tail. But in the typical patient the left lobe of the liver is small, so when we try to do this, we reach the point where the scan plane moves off the left lobe and onto the stomach, and our image disappears. We lose not only the pancreas but the splenic vein as well.

Look at Figure 10–11. Line A on this diagram represents the longitudinal scan plane in the midline—the one that produces pictures like

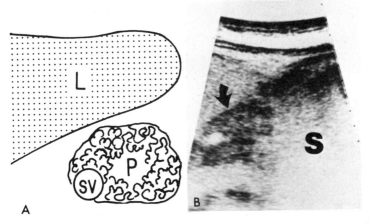

Figure 10–10. Longitudinal scans through the left lobe of the liver give good images of the body of the pancreas.

A. A diagramatic representation of the anatomy. L = liver, P = pancreas, SV = splenic vein.

B. A longitudinal scan in the midline showing the liver, splenic vein, and pancreas (*arrow*). Notice the large shadow cast by air in the bowel (S).

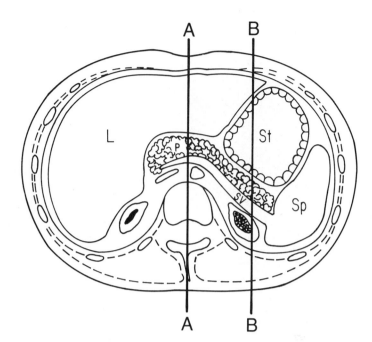

Figure 10–11. This diagram shows two possible longitudinal scan planes. See text for explanation.

Figure 10–10. If we moved the scanner to the patient's left until the scan plane was at a position marked by line B, the sound beam would be traversing the stomach and we would have lost our acoustic window and could no longer see the pancreas.

Now look at Figure 10–12. Here again line A represents the midline longitudinal scan plane that produces a nice picture of the pancreas. But instead of sliding the scanner to the left as we did in the previous diagram, suppose we slide the scanner to the patient's *right* and then angle it so that the sound beam passes along the path marked by line C. If we do this, we will still have a good picture of the pancreas. We have kept the scan plane passing through the liver as an acoustic window and have adjusted the scan angle so that the sound beam is now passing through the body and tail of the pancreas. (Now you can see why we describe

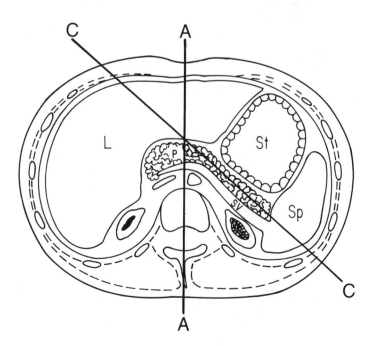

Figure 10–12. This diagram shows the correct scan plane for a "down-the-tail" view of the pancreas. See text for explanation.

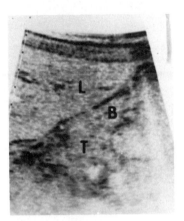

Figure 10–13. By using the liver for an acoustic window and angling the scan plane it is possible to see "down the tail" of the pancreas. See the text and Figure 10–12 for orientation. L = liver, B = body of pancreas, T = tail of pancreas.

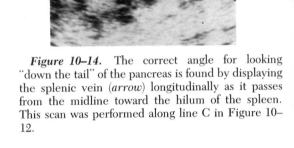

Figure 10–14. The correct angle for looking "down the tail" of the pancreas is found by displaying the splenic vein (*arrow*) longitudinally as it passes from the midline toward the hilum of the spleen. This scan was performed along line C in Figure 10–12.

this view as looking "down the tail" of the pancreas.) Figure 10–13 is a "down-the-tail" scan of a normal pancreas. Refer back to Figure 10–12 for orientation. Remember that we are looking at both the body and the tail of the pancreas on the same image; the portion of the gland that is closest to the skin surface is the body, and as the sound beam moves deeper it passes through the tail

It sounds simple, you say, but how do I find the correct scan angle to look down the tail? Remember that the pancreas very closely follows the splenic vein, and the splenic vein is easy to see because it is echo-free. Begin your scan in a midline longitudinal section, which is easy to obtain (Figure 10–10). Keep watching the splenic vein and begin tilting the scan plane toward the left. Your goal is to tilt the scan plane until the splenic vein is visible lengthwise passing from just beneath the liver down into the spleen as shown in Figure 10–14. As you increase the angle, you will find that you have to move the scanner to the patient's *right*; failure to do this usually results in a sudden loss of the picture as the sound beam passes through the stomach. If you are increasing the scan angle to look down the tail of the pancreas and the splenic vein suddenly disappears from view it means you must move the scanner more to the right to avoid the stomach.

It takes careful adjustment and fine tuning of

the scan plane to get the precise entrance point and scan angle for seeing the tail of the pancreas clearly. Again, the flexibility of the real-time scanner is important; down-the-tail views are excruciatingly difficult and frustrating with a manual scanner. With the real-time machine we can see the entire body and tail of the pancreas in about 85 per cent of our patients.

PATHOLOGIC APPEARANCE

Size

Pancreatic enlargement may be either generalized (involving the entire gland) or focal. Generalized pancreatic enlargement occurs only in **acute pancreatitis**, and when the organ is uniformly big, this diagnosis should be suggested. What is too big? Certainly any gland more than 3 cm thick is enlarged; and when the thickness approaches 2.5 cm, we begin to get suspicious. As we said earlier, however, there is considerable variability in the size of the pancreas, so the ultrasonologist must learn to relate the size of the pancreas to the size of the patient. While 3 cm represents enlargement in anyone, 2 cm may be too large in a thin, 70 pound fashion model.

All this may sound like terribly confusing business, but it is not actually so difficult in

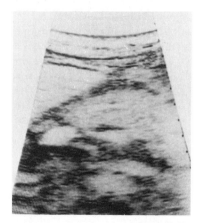

Figure 10–15. Acute pancreatitis can cause the pancreas to enlarge and its echo texture to decrease. In addition the pancreatic duct is dilated in this patient. Transverse section.

practice. When the pancreas is enlarged, it stands out like a sore thumb; it is easy to scan in almost any orientation and looks like a large bratwurst draped over the spinal column (Figure 10–15). This appearance is almost pathognomonic for acute pancreatitis. There are only two other conditions that can mimic this finding: enlarged retroperitoneal lymph nodes and a horseshoe kidney.

Texture

When the echo intensity in the pancreas is less than that of the adjacent liver, it is abnormal. (Of course, we must first be certain that the echo intensity of the liver is not abnormally increased; this is easily done by comparing the liver echoes with those of the kidney, as we saw in Chapter 8.) There is only one diagnosis to consider when the echo texture of the pancreas is less than that of the liver: **acute** or "**subacute**" **pancreatitis.** Usually the pancreas will also be enlarged in this disease; this makes the diagnosis even more certain (see Figure 10–15). Sometimes in patients with acute pancreatitis the texture is normal; ultrasound, therefore, is *not useful* in *excluding* the diagnosis of acute pancreatitis.

Frontiers of medicine department: It is generally accepted that the sine qua non for the diagnosis of acute pancreatitis is an elevated blood amylase level. Over the past few years we have observed a group of patients, predominantly young women in their twenties, who have all the clinical features of mild pancreatitis but in whom we have not been able to document an elevation of the blood amylase level. The pancreas in all of these patients has been enlarged, with echo intensities less than those of the liver. The symptoms resolved in three to six months, and after that time the pancreas had a more normal appearance on the ultrasound scan. We call this "subacute" pancreatitis, and the diagnosis rests on demonstrating an enlarged and relatively echo-free pancreas in the presence of normal blood amylase levels. This is not a widely accepted clinical diagnosis, but our clinicians agree that the signs and symptoms point to pancreatitic disease and agree with the ultrasonic findings.

Most ultrasonologists believe that the pathologic condition of **chronic pancreatitis** produces an increase in the intensity of the pancreatic echoes. While this is undoubtedly true, there is no reliable way to detect increased pancreatic echogenicity with ultrasound. Remember that the normal pancreas can be very echogenic because of nonpathologic fatty infiltration. There is no way to differentiate this appearance from that of chronic pancreatitis. On rare occasions it may be possible to demonstrate calcifications with shadowing in the pancreas, and when such calcifications are present, the diagnosis of chronic pancreatitis can be confidently entertained. In the absence of calcifications, however, the diagnosis must rest on clinical grounds. (A further clue to the diagnosis of chronic pancreatitis is the presence of ductal dilatation.)

Pancreatic Duct

You already know our opinion on the pancreatic duct; if the lumen of the duct is visible, it is abnormal. The duct becomes dilated when it is **obstructed** by **gallstones** or a **tumor,** or when there is long-standing **periductal inflammation** and scarring. Figure 10–16 shows a dilated pancreatic duct. Obstruction of the pancreatic duct causes acute pancreatitis in the remainder of the organ, and the subsequent decrease in echogenicity and enlargement of the gland make the dilated duct even more prominent. One must be careful not to confuse the hepatic artery or the back wall of the stomach with the pancreatic duct. You will never make this mistake as long as you remember that the pancreatic duct runs within pancreatic tissue; make certain that the structure you plan to call the duct has pancreas both above (ventral to) and below (dorsal to) it.

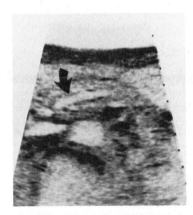

Figure 10–16. When the pancreatic duct is obstructed it enlarges (*arrow*). An obstructing gallstone has caused the pancreatic duct and its side branches to dilate in this patient. Transverse section.

Focal Solid Mass

Whenever there is a focal area of pancreatic enlargement it must be considered pathologic; if there is any alteration in the echo texture in the enlarged area it is definitely pathologic.

For all intents and purposes there is only one thing that causes a focal solid mass in the pancreas: **pancreatic carcinoma** (Figure 10–17). Once in a blue moon you may encounter a **nonpancreatic tumor** metastatic to a local lymph node, **a pancreatic islet cell tumor,** or an unusual form of **focal pancreatitis.** In general, it is wisest to call all focal solid lesions carcinoma until they are proved otherwise. Tumors may be very small. Figure 10–17C is a small carcinoma in the body of the pancreas. We correctly diagnosed this case from the ultrasound appearance because of the subtle, but real, difference in echo texture in the lesion. Be very careful in scrutinizing the pancreas and be prepared to call any suspicious focal enlargement or any area of altered echo texture abnormal. The patient with such findings deserves further evaluation (such as a CT scan, percutaneous biopsy, or even laparotomy).

Focal Mass With Cystic Areas

Figure 10–18 shows a focal mass in the pancreas that contains some echo-free or cystic areas. Even though such a lesion could represent carcinoma, in our experience this is no longer the most likely diagnosis. Cystic areas in the pancreas should always suggest a complication of pancreatitis: **phlegmon** or **evolving pseudocyst.** Acute pancreatitis can resolve in several ways. Most commonly the inflammation subsides and the pancreas returns to its normal, preinflammation appearance. Sometimes, however, one or more areas of the pancreas may undergo necrosis and not heal with the rest of

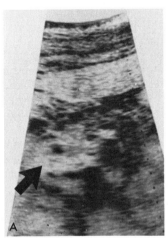
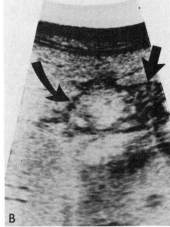
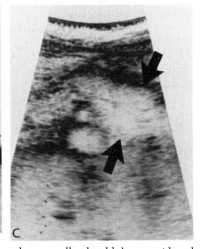

Figure 10–17. Any focal solid mass in the pancreas, no matter how small, should be considered carcinoma until proved otherwise.

A. A carcinoma with decreased echoes is seen in the head of the pancreas (*arrow*). Transverse section.

B. Although this cancer (*curved arrow*) is less than 3 cm in size, it is easily recognized because it is larger than the rest of the pancreas (*straight arrow*) and has an altered echo texture. Transverse section.

C. Even subtle focal masses (*arrows*) should be considered carcinoma. Transverse section.

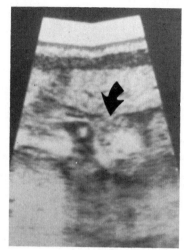

Figure 10–18. Focal masses with cystic areas (*arrow*) should suggest phlegmon—a focal area of destruction secondary to pancreatitis. This is a phlegmon in the tail of the pancreas seen in transverse section.

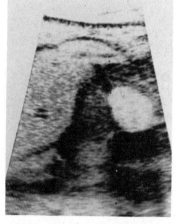

Figure 10–19. Focal cystic masses in the pancreas are pseudocysts. This longitudinal scan demonstrates a pseudocyst in the head of the pancreas.

the gland. This results in a focal area of gland inflammation known as a "phlegmon." The patient usually has persistent symptoms of pancreatitis and will usually have an elevated blood amylase level. Sometimes pancreatitis heals slowly; the local mass subsides, and the cystic areas are replaced with normal pancreatic echoes. In other cases the inflammatory process may persist, and the necrosis may become more widespread until the entire area has become liquefied and cystic. When this happens, the patient has developed a pseudocyst.

Focal Cystic Mass

When a cystic mass is identified within the pancreas, the only diagnosis to consider is **pseudocyst** (Figure 10–19). Pseudocysts are common complications of pancreatitis. They represent walled-off accumulations of pancreatic juices and vary greatly in size and location. Once a pseudocyst has formed, it often can grow to quite a large size and may spread widely throughout the abdomen. Pseudocyst is an easy ultrasonic diagnosis to make provided it is modest in size and can be recognized as arising from the pancreas. When there is more than one pseudocyst, when the pseudocyst contains internal septations, or when the pseudocyst becomes very large and dissects into other organs or other areas of the abdomen, the diagnosis may be more difficult. A very useful rule is to

consider all cystic lesions that appear in the region of the pancreas to be pseudocysts. The clinical presentation will usually verify your impression.

The only condition that you are likely to confuse with pseudocyst is **lymphoma**. Remember that lymphoma can be well circumscribed and echo-free and that there are lymph nodes in the region of the pancreas. Lymphoma in these nodes could be easily confused with a pseudocyst (or acute pancreatitis) on the basis of the ultrasound appearance. Frequently, however, the through transmission of sound will not be as great with lymphoma as with pseudocyst. Also the clinical presentation of these diseases is quite different and should enable you to make a correct diagnosis.

PERSPECTIVE

The pancreas is a challenging but rewarding organ for ultrasound study. It will require some practice before you feel comfortable in recognizing this organ and even longer before you have a good eye for what is normal and what is abnormal. Once you have paid your dues, however, you will find that pancreatic diagnosis is reasonably straightforward; there are few disease processes that effect the gland and they have fairly characteristic ultrasonic appearances.

BIBLIOGRAPHY

Filly, R. A., and London, L. S.: The normal pancreas: acoustic characteristics and frequency of imaging. *Journal of Clinical Ultrasound* 7:121 (1979).
(This paper discusses the echogenicity and texture of the normal pancreas.)

Arger, P. H., Mulhern, C. B., Bonavita, J. A., et al.: An analysis of pancreatic sonography in suspected pancreatic disease. *Journal of Clinical Ultrasound* 7:91 (1979).
(This analysis of 500 patients provides mountains of numerical data and pancreatic measurements.)

Laing, F. C., Gooding, G. A. W., Brown, T., et al.: Atypical pseudocysts of the pancreas: an ultrasonic evaluation. *Journal of Clinical Ultrasound* 7:27 (1979).
(Pseudocysts can be deceptive, as this paper points out.)

Taylor, K. J. W., Buchin, P. J., Viscorni, G. N., et al.: Ultrasonic scanning of the pancreas. *Radiology* 138:211 (1981).
(CT scanners can't possibly handle the numbers of patients with potential pancreatic disease; ultrasound will have a big role for many years to come. This paper tells why.)

Chapter 11

THE KIDNEYS AND PARARENAL AREAS

Kidneys

The evaluation of mass lesions in the kidneys was among the first important uses of ultrasound in the abdomen. Years ago, using equipment that was primitive beyond belief, early pioneers in ultrasound were able to separate renal tumors from renal cysts with reasonable accuracy. They could not tell much else in those days, but this ability to provide reliable diagnostic information about a common problem was an important first step in the evolution of abdominal ultrasonography as we know it today. As the years have gone by, however, it has become clear that despite the fact that the kidneys are a rather simple morphologic system, afflicted with only a limited number of diseases, renal ultasound is not easy. The organs themselves are usually tough to image in their entirety, and it can be surprisingly difficult to differentiate a renal cyst from a tumor. Expertise in renal ultrasound comes only after lots of practice on patients.

NORMAL APPEARANCE

Anatomy

The kidneys are, well . . . kidney-shaped. They lie in the posterior half of both sides of the abdomen separated from the spine by the psoas muscles. The kidneys are retroperitoneal and are surrounded and cushioned by a layer of fat. The right kidney is covered anteriorly by the right lobe of the liver and, because of the liver's bulk, is usually 2 or 3 cm farther caudad than the left. The stomach and the colon lie in front of (anterior to) the left kidney. The spleen is positioned lateral and slightly dorsal to the upper pole of the left kidney. Usually each kidney has one artery and one vein that run directly from the adjacent aorta and inferior vena cava (see Chapter 6); these vessels enter the hilum of the kidney and then branch to

distribute and receive blood from the renal parenchyma. (About 20 per cent of patients have more than one artery to each kidney, but it is usually not possible to determine this from the ultrasound images.)

The kidney itself is divided into two major anatomic areas: the renal parenchyma and the renal sinus. The renal parenchyma contains the functional tissue of the kidney. It forms the outer part of the organ and is made up of several complex types of cells. For ultrasound purposes it is only necessary to distinguish between the renal cortex and the medulla. The cortex contains the renal glomeruli and proximal renal tubule loops, while the medulla is made up of the radially oriented loops of Henle and the distal tubules. We need not delve more deeply into the complexities of renal anatomy and physiology; it is enough for us to know that the renal cortex makes up the bulk of the renal parenchyma and that the renal medullae are small pyramids located on the inner aspect of the parenchyma with their apices directed toward the renal sinus. The renal sinus is the central portion of the kidney that contains the collecting system (the calyces, infundibula, and pelvis) as well as the major branches of the renal artery and vein. All the structures in the sinus are surrounded by fat, which increases in thickness with age and in many disease states. Figure 11–1 is a scan of a normal kidney.

Size

The kidneys are somewhat variable in size. They average 10 to 13 cm in length and 4 to 6 cm in greatest width. The left kidney is slightly larger than the right in most patients. The renal outline is usually smooth and continuous, but occasionally there will be focal "humps" in the contour that are normal and are caused by the way the kidney is formed embryologically. They are commonly known as "fetal lobulations."

119

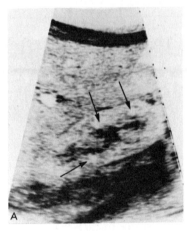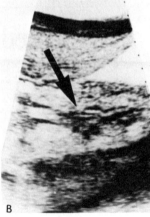

Figure 11–1. The normal kidney is composed of parenchyma and renal sinus.

A. The echo texture of the renal parenchyma is normally less than the liver. In some patients the renal pyramids or medullae can be identified as areas of slightly decreased echogenicity within the parenchyma *(arrows)*.

B. The renal sinus *(arrow)* is composed of many different tissues and it therefore is highly echogenic. Portions of the renal arteries, veins, and collecting system are often seen.

Regardless of the contour of the kidney, the renal parenchyma should have a uniform thickness. If there is a bump or hump in the renal contour, there should also be a corresponding bump in the underlying renal sinus (Figure 11–2). The width of the renal parenchyma is between 1 and 2 cm in the midportions of the organ and 2 and 3 cm at the poles.

Sometimes the kidney appears to be made up of two smaller units that have fused together. This condition is known as a "partial duplication" and is accompanied by a double, or "bifid," collecting system. In some scan planes this type of kidney will appear to have two separate renal sinuses separated by an island of normal renal parenchyma (Figure 11–3).

Texture

The renal parenchyma is not highly echogenic; its echo levels are normally lower than those of the liver. In many normal patients it is possible to distinguish the cortical and medullary components of the renal parenchyma because the medullae are even less echogenic than the renal cortex (see Figure 11–1). If the cortical and medullary tissue can be distinguished, the difference in texture should always be very slight. If this difference is marked, it usually indicates renal disease, as we shall see in a moment.

The renal sinus is made up of very heterogeneous tissues—fat, vessel and collecting system walls, urine in the lumen of the collecting system, and blood in the vessels. It is, therefore, an area of high-intensity echoes interrupted by occasional sections of tubular structures, whose echo-free lumens represent the

major intrarenal vessels or portions of the collecting system, as shown in Figure 11–1.

SCANNING TECHNIQUE

Before the advent of real-time the kidneys were traditionally scanned with the patient in the prone position, and the thick muscles of the back were used as an acoustic window. Somehow things never went as smoothly as they should; there always seemed to be some part of the kidney that could not be well demonstrated. Real-time scanners, offering more flexibility in scan plane, revealed new and better acoustic windows.

We believe that the right kidney is best seen by using the right lobe of the liver as an acoustic window. If the liver is large, it may be possible

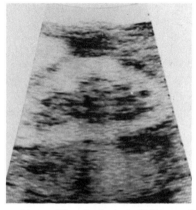

Figure 11–2. The thickness of the renal parenchyma should be constant; if there is a "bump" in the cortex there should also be a "bump" in the sinus underneath it.

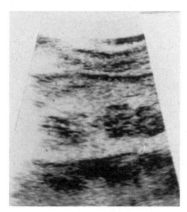

Figure 11–3. Partial duplication of the kidney causes relative separation of the renal sinus echoes in some scan planes.

to scan through the anterior abdominal wall with the patient supine. In most cases, however, it is necessary to move the scan plane over toward the patient's flank to use a frontal (coronal) scan plane; the resulting view of the kidney resembles that with which we are familiar from intravenous urography. The transducer should be as far toward the patient's feet as possible while still keeping over the right lobe of the liver; this will minimize shadows due to the ribs. If the right lobe of the liver is so small that it cannot be brought out from underneath the rib cage in deep inspiration, we often turn the patient up onto his left side and sometimes drape him over a pillow to stretch out the right flank. The scanner must be moved even farther posteriorly so that the kidney is seen from below (caudad to) the lowest rib. Only rarely is it necessary to turn the patient prone and bring the sound beam in from the back; if you are forced to try this, then the ball game is probably over.

There is no acoustic window like the liver to let you see the left kidney from the front of the body. The spleen, however, lies along the lateral and posterior aspect of the kidney and sometimes can provide access for the sound beam. The patient will have to be turned onto his right side, and the transducer must be placed near the midaxillary line or slightly dorsal to it. As with the right kidney, scan planes that are approximately frontal sections are generally the most useful. The transducer may have to be moved craniad so that it rests over or between the ribs. In this position there will almost always be rib shadows in the image, creating a "venetian blind" effect. The sonographer must look through the openings in the

"venetian blind" and keep his attention concentrated on the parts of the kidney that are visible. By having the patient control respiration it is usually possible to bring all of the kidney into view.

In general we prefer to perform kidney scans in sections both parallel and perpendicular to the long axis of the kidney. Scanning in both planes is necessary to avoid overlooking subtle lesions that may project outside the general outline of the kidney, particularly anteriorly or posteriorly.

PATHOLOGIC APPEARANCE

Size

In theory there are a variety of disease processes that cause diffuse enlargement of the kidneys: **acute pyelonephritis, acute glomerulonephritis,** various **metabolic storage diseases,** diffusely **infiltrative tumors** such as **lymphoma** and **polycystic disease.** In actual practice, enlargement of the kidneys is rare. The commonest condition you are likely to encounter causing enlargement of the kidneys is polycystic disease (and in this case the multiple cysts make the diagnosis easy).

You will, however, frequently find small kidneys (anything less than 9 cm is "small" to us). When renal parenchyma decreases, there may be a concomitant increase in the renal sinus; so that while the overall renal size is not noticeably below normal, the ratio of parenchyma to sinus is decreased. Almost any kind of **chronic renal disease** will produce a uniformly small kidney; **glomerular disease** (including Kimmelstiel-Wilson disease in diabetes), chronic **renal ischemia, chronic pyelonephritis,** and **nephrosclerosis** all lead to diminished renal parenchyma, small kidneys, and enlarged renal sinuses.

Sometimes the loss of renal tissue occurs in a focal manner so that one part of the kidney is normal in size but another is small or shrunken. Either localized **chronic pyelonephritis** or prior **ischemic infarcts** can produce this appearance.

Texture

As with the increased renal size, there are several pathologic processes that can cause edema of the renal parenchyma and hence decease its echogenicity. These include **acute pyelonephritis, acute glomerulonephritis, ob-**

struction, and **acute ischemic injury.** We have found it difficult in practice to recognize these conditions. The changes are subtle; and if you are to recognize them, close correlation with clinical findings is necessary. Just as the renal atrophy of chronic disease leads to an increase in size of the renal sinuses, those conditions that cause swelling decrease the size of the sinuses, and the strong central echoes look as though they are being "squeezed."

It is much easier to recognize when the renal parenchymal echoes are abnormally increased. Increased echogenicity occurs in a variety of disease processes, all of which involve abnormalities of the cortex; and for the most part, the disease processes appear to be those that lead to interstitial rather than glomerular abnormalities. At present we do not attempt a specific diagnosis; we simply mention that the renal cortical echoes are diffusely increased and this indicates a diffuse disease process in the renal parenchyma.

There are two ways to determine whether there is increased echogenicity of the renal parenchyma. The first is to compare the intensity of the renal cortical echoes with the liver echoes. The echo intensity of the liver should always be greater than that of the renal cortex. If the renal cortical echoes are equal to or greater than those in the liver, there is diffuse renal disease. Second, because the renal medullae do not change their echogenicity in these processes, they will stand out more clearly as the renal cortical echoes increase. Any time the cortical-medullary definition is unusually prominent, the possibility of diffuse renal cortical disease should be considered (Figure 11–4). Because cortical-medullary differentiation is subjective, we always verify any impression of abnormality by comparing the renal and hepatic echoes.

Cystic Focal Lesions

Cysts in the renal parenchyma are a dime a dozen; about 15 per cent of our patients have at least one and sometimes several renal cysts, and the frequency seems to increase with age. It is neither possible nor desirable to perform cyst punctures or arteriography on all these patients; therefore, it is important to have a good idea of what constitutes a benign cyst. There are three commonly accepted criteria. First, a renal cyst should contain no internal echoes. Second, the inner walls of a benign cyst should be smooth and uniform. Finally, there should be acoustic enhancement in the tissues beyond a cyst.

As is so often the case in the application of such simply stated rules, it is uncommon to find a cyst that fulfills all three of these criteria. Spurious "echoes" often appear in the middle of cysts. These are due to any of a variety of artifacts, which we discussed in Chapter 4. Even when some low-level signals are present in a cyst, however, it is usually possible to demonstrate a difference between its echogenicity and that of the immediately adjacent renal parenchyma. Except in very small cysts, it should be possible to demonstrate a smooth, continuous posterior wall; and we have found that this is the most constant sign of a benign cystic lesion. Acoustic enhancement can often be difficult to appreciate on the ultrasound image. In the scan planes that show the kidney best there may be gas-bearing bowel immediately beyond the renal image, and the shadows and reverberations generated there can distort the acoustic enhancement and make it difficult to recognize. Here again, however, real-time has proved to be helpful in finding a scan plane that shows enhancement. Figure 11–5 shows examples of renal cysts.

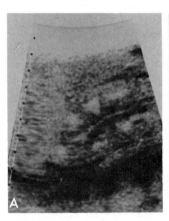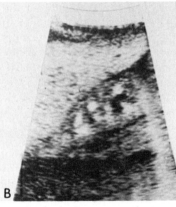

Figure 11–4. Many diffuse diseases of the renal cortex cause an increase in its echogenicity. The medulla becomes very prominent, and the cortical echoes may be more intense than those of the liver.

A. Diabetic nephropathy (Kimmelstiel-Wilson kidney).

B. Acute glomerulonephritis in a child.

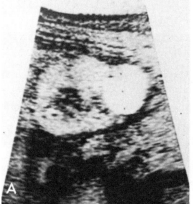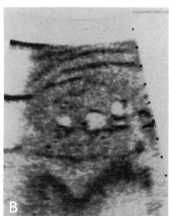

Figure 11–5. Renal cysts should be echo-free, have a smooth posterior wall, and show acoustic enhancement.
  A. A moderate size renal cyst.
  B. Three small parapelvic cysts.

There is a large body of literature discussing the etiology and the significance of renal cysts, and it is beyond the scope of this book to rehash this in any detail. The important thing to remember is that the overwhelming majority of cystic lesions are benign and of no consequence to the patient.

Primum non nocere department: Ironically, the greatest danger to the patient posed by a renal cyst may be that the "health care team" will become unduly excited about the discovery of the cyst and inflict aggressive diagnostic and sometimes "therapeutic" torture on the hapless patient.

There are several syndromes in which multiple renal cysts do, however, have significant medical problems associated with them. The only one that is common is **polycystic kidney disease.** These patients have many cysts in both kidneys, and these cysts vary greatly in size. The kidneys are usually enlarged overall, and there may be associated cysts in the liver. This is a serious congenital condition that ultimately progresses to renal failure, and one that is important to recognize.

Solid Focal Lesions

For all practical purposes, there is only one benign solid focal lesion of the kidney—the **column of Bertin**, a double layer of renal cortex that is folded in toward the center of the kidney, displacing a portion of the renal sinus (Figure 11–6). The echo texture is *exactly the same* as the adjacent renal cortex, and the width of the "mass" is twice as great as the adjacent renal cortical thickness. Because the column of Bertin is a common normal anatomic variant, the ul-

trasonographer must learn to recognize it with confidence. Fortunately, the appearance is characteristic (if you have seen one, you have seen them all, as they say), so almost always a column of Bertin can be differentiated from other kinds of solid abnormalities.

Any other focal solid masses or lesions in the kidneys are **carcinoma** until proved otherwise (and it is not often that they are proved otherwise). There is a rare condition known as **focal interstitial nephritis** that appears as a solid focal mass. This is actually an acute renal infection and is probably best considered as a renal abscess without any liquefaction. There are also occasional benign tumors of the kidneys such as an **angiomyolipoma.** Because in many cases there is no reliable way of differentiating these

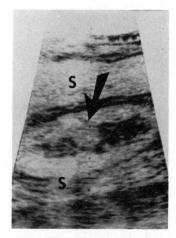

Figure 11–6. The column of Bertin (*arrow*) has two characteristics: Its echogenicity is identical to that of the renal cortex, and its width is twice that of the renal cortex. Notice the acoustic shadow cast by the twelfth rib (S).

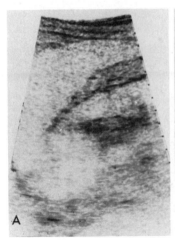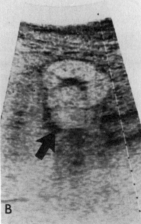

Figure 11–7. Solid focal lesions that enlarge the renal cortex are nearly always carcinoma.

lesions ultrasonically from the much more common carcinoma, carcinoma must be the primary diagnosis when a focal solid lesion of the kidney is found (Figure 11–7).

Mixed Focal Lesions

A focal renal lesion that contains some cystic elements but does not fulfill the criteria for a benign renal cyst is considered a mixed (or complex) mass. In the kidney such lesions are either **carcinoma** or **abscess**, and we do not know of any way to distinguish the two on the basis of the ultrasound appearance. Usually the clinical setting is helpful; and, for this reason, it is not likely that you will make a diagnostic error. If there are any diagnostic uncertainties, it is an easy matter to perform a percutaneous biopsy to establish the correct diagnosis.

Renal Sinus

We have already referred to the enlargement of the renal sinus that accompanies the loss of renal parenchyma. It is important to remember, however, that as a normal component of the aging process we all slowly lose renal parenchymal cells that are replaced by fat cells in the renal sinus; the sinus *normally* enlarges with advancing age. In some people this process is quite pronounced and leads to a very large renal sinus with greatly thinned renal parenchyma (Figure 11–8). This enlargement of the sinus is known as **renal sinus fibrolipomatosis**. Despite the rather impressive name this condition is not usually of clinical significance to the patient.

Stones in the renal collecting system look just like stones in the gallbladder: They produce high-intensity echoes and cast shadows (Figure 11–9). Although this is a dramatic ultrasound finding, we still consider intravenous urography to be the primary method of evaluating calculous disease of the kidneys and the urinary tract.

The most important pathologic condition of the renal sinus is **hydronephrosis**. When the flow of urine is obstructed, the renal collecting systems become enlarged and can be recognized as echo-free structures in the center of the renal sinus (Figure 11–10). In its earliest stages hydronephrosis can be difficult to recognize. As the dilatation worsens, however, the infundibula may dilate and project into the renal parenchyma, and the renal pelvis enlarges. In very severe hydronephrosis the enlargement

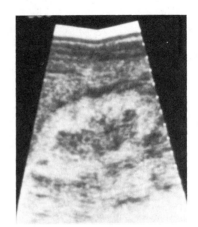

Figure 11–8. Renal sinus fibrolipomatosis is the slow enlargement of the renal sinus that occurs with advancing age.

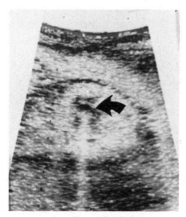

Figure 11–9. Stones in the kidney or renal pelvis (*arrow*) cast shadows just as do stones or calcifications elsewhere.

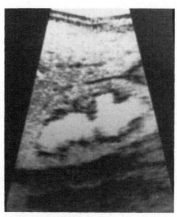

Figure 11–10. Hydronephrosis is dilatation of the renal pelvis and calyces. It produces an oblong cystic area within the renal sinus.

may be so great that the renal parenchyma is thinned and sometimes is barely perceptible.

Hydronephrosis is a fairly straightforward ultrasound diagnosis, but there are a few things to watch out for. (1) Do not be fooled by prominent cortical-medullary differentiation. In renal cortical disease the medullae often appear as cystic areas, which should not be mistaken for hydronephrosis. Remember that hydronephrosis is a process that affects the renal sinus, while the medullae are located in the renal parenchyma. (2) Normal, extrarenal pelvises located outside the renal sinus are common anatomic variants (Figure 11–11). (3) Sometimes peripelvic cysts are multiple and simulate an enlarged collecting system. If hydronephrosis is truly present, however, the pelvis itself should be easily seen and should serve as an important differentiating point. In all cases of hydronephrosis the sonographer should try to follow the dilatation of the collecting system as far down the ureter as possible in an attempt to delineate the site of obstruction. If the proximal ureter is dilated, the diagnosis of obstructive uropathy is clear. Because the ureter is frequently obscured by overlying bowel, however, you will find the site of obstruction in only about 25 per cent of cases. Even if you have not located the block, you have done the patient a genuine service by identifying the presence of obstruction quickly and without the use of contrast agent.

Spleen

The spleen is traditionally discussed in the liver chapter. From an ultrasonic point of view,

however, it has little in common with the liver; and because it is best scanned in the same planes as the left kidney, we have chosen to discuss it here. The scanning techniques are essentially the same as for the left kidney. You will have to turn the patient onto his right side and scan over or through the ribs. The spleen is approximately the same size as the left kidney, but has none of the strong central echoes. It is normally very homogeneous, and the echoes within it are of the same intensity as the renal cortex (i.e., slightly lower-level than those in the liver).

The spleen is often enlarged, and there are

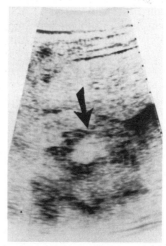

Figure 11–11. Sometimes the renal pelvis lies outside the renal sinus as shown in this transverse scan of the right kidney. These "extra-renal pelves" (*arrow*) are larger than normal and must not be mistaken for hydronephrosis.

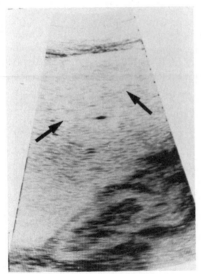

Figure 11–12. The spleen is enlarged when it measures more than 12 cm or is larger than the kidney. This patient has leukemia: Notice the focal areas of splenic necrosis (*arrows*).

two ways to recognize this. First, if any single dimension of the spleen is greater than 12 cm, it should be considered enlarged. Second, if the overall volume of the spleen is greater than that of the left kidney, the spleen is enlarged (assuming, of course, that the kidney itself is normal). We have never been successful at differentiating the various conditions that produce splenomegaly on the basis of the echo texture of the spleen, except to recognize an occasional benign splenic cyst or other focal lesion (Figure 11–12).

Conditions that produce focal abnormalities in the spleen include **metastases, infarcts,** and **granulomatous infections** (TB, histoplasmosis, and the like). Infarcts and granulomas sometimes—but certainly not always—calcify and cast a shadow. Usually there is no way to make a specific diagnosis from the ultrasound scan. Fortunately the clinical data are often sufficient to permit a precise diagnosis.

Finally a word about splenic trauma. The spleen is easily injured by blunt abdominal trauma, and this can produce either a local disruption of the spleen with hemorrhage or a crescent-shaped hematoma just under the splenic capsule (Figure 11–13). While these conditions can sometimes be visualized on ultrasound scans, there has not been much interest in our laboratory (or elsewhere) for using ultrasound to assess the spleen in trauma. The problem is that these patients are usually diffi-

cult to examine because of pain in the left upper quadrant of the abdomen, and consequently there are frequent false negative examinations. Other imaging procedures such as radionuclide scan, CT scan, or angiography are better for this problem.

Adrenals

The adrenals are small, thin, pyramid-shaped glands that usually sit like dunce caps atop the upper poles of the kidneys. They are between 1 and 3 cm in size, easily within the resolution capabilities of modern scanners. Unfortunately, the normal adrenals are very difficult to recognize with certainty. Even though some authors feel comfortable saying that they can see the normal glands, we have never felt we could do so reliably.

Chutzpah department: It is always possible to point to some wedge-shaped area adjacent to the kidney and say in a loud authoritative voice, "There is the adrenal!" Nobody will argue with you, but are you really correct?

Whether or not one can see normal adrenals makes little difference, because most pathologic conditions cause them to enlarge. When the glands are enlarged, it is easy to see them, and you will have no trouble provided you remember to look for them (Figure 11–14). Unfortunately, there is no way to differentiate among the various types of benign and malignant tu-

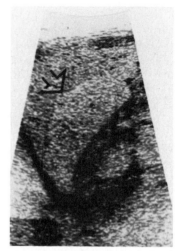

Figure 11–13. A splenic hematoma (*arrow*) has a different echo texture from the remainder of the spleen.

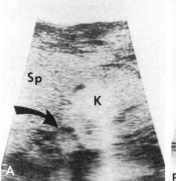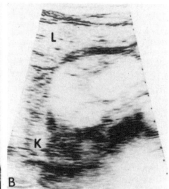

Figure 11–14. If the adrenal glands are easy to see they are enlarged.

A. A prominent left adrenal gland (*arrow*) in a patient with adrenal hyperplasia. Sp = spleen, K = kidney.

B. A large, complex carcinoma of the right adrenal gland. L = liver, K = kidney.

mors that affect the adrenals on the basis of the appearance of the ultrasound scan alone.

Adrenal ultrasonography is actually quite easy. Any scan plane that will enable you to see the upper poles of the kidneys can be used. The whole trick is in remembering to look for them near the upper poles of the kidneys while keeping these rules in mind: (1) If you cannot definitely find the adrenal glands, they are almost certainly normal. (2) If an adrenal can be easily seen, it is almost certainly enlarged and abnormal. (3) There is no ultrasonic way of making a specific pathologic diagnosis if an adrenal mass is encountered.

Retroperitoneum

The retroperitoneal space extends from above the upper poles of the kidneys down to the pelvis, and the sonographer will sometimes encounter pathologic processes in this area. As is the case in any other organ or area of the body, these lesions are either cystic, solid, or mixed.

Cystic lesions are uncommon. Occasionally an acute hemorrhage will appear cystic for a few hours and might be found following trauma. A rupture of part of the urinary collecting system may cause a localized collection of urine (a urinoma) to form, a problem that is usually a complication of surgery. Much more common than truly cystic lesions are masses of malignant lymphoma that simulate cysts. Recall from Chapter 7 that any type of lymphoma can be echo-poor and is easily mistaken for a cyst. The retroperitoneal space is liberally supplied with lymph nodes, and lymphoma is a fairly common disease; therefore, whenever you see what appears to be a cystic lesion in the retroperitoneum, lymphoma should come immediately to mind.

Solid or echogenic masses in the retroperitoneum are most commonly malignant tumors, either metastatic carcinoma or sarcoma. Occasionally an old hematoma or an abscess will contain echoes, and once in your lifetime you may encounter a case of retroperitoneal fibrosis. Statistically, a tumor is the most likely possibility, and it should always be your first diagnostic suggestion. It is an easy matter to verify the diagnosis with a percutaneous biopsy.

Finally, there are several causes for mixed or complex lesions of the retroperitoneum. The commonest of these is retroperitoneal abscess. Occasionally, large retroperitoneal tumors have necrotic fluid-filled centers that will be echo-free, and retroperitoneal hematomas might present as a mixture of echogenic and echo-free areas.

BIBLIOGRAPHY

Rosenfield, A. T., Taylor, K. J. W., Crade, M., et al.: Anatomy and pathology of the kidney by gray-scale ultrasound. *Radiology 128*:737 (1978).
(A well-illustrated discussion of intrarenal anatomy and general pathology. The authors introduce "Type I" and "Type II" renal disease. Read "diffuse" for "Type I" and "focal" for "Type II" and you won't get confused.)

Lee, J. K. T., McClennan, B. L., Nelson, G. L., et al.: Acute focal bacterial nephritis. *American Journal of Roentgenology* 135:87 (1980).
(This is a good discussion of this rare disease—a focal lesion in the kidney secondary to infection.)

Silver, T. M., Campbell, D., Wicks, J. D., et al.: Peritransplant fluid collections. *Radiology* 138:145 (1981).
(This is the most recent discussion of the various complications of renal transplants.)

Rosenfield, A. T., Taylor, K. J. W., Dembner, A. G., et al.: Ultrasound of the renal sinus. *American Journal of Roentgenology* 133:441 (1979).
(More than you want to know about the renal sinus.)

Chapter 12

THE PELVIS

Yes, we know that the pelvis is actually an anatomic area rather than a single organ system; however, we see no reason to depart from time-honored convention and will, therefore, stretch our organ orientation to discuss the pelvic organs all together. First we will deal with the female pelvis and, because clinical problems and pathologic conditions of this region are quite different in the pregnant and the nonpregnant states, we have divided our discussion along these lines: first the nonpregnant pelvis, then ultrasound scanning in early pregnancy—the first 12 weeks of gestation. We do not want to be accused of sex discrimination, so you will find at the end of the chapter a brief discussion of ultrasound findings in the male pelvis.

Female Pelvis

NORMAL APPEARANCE
Anatomy

The uterus is a pear-shaped organ that lies in the midline, immediately beneath the posterior wall of the bladder. The narrow neck is called the **cervix,** the central section the **body,** and the bulbous end the **fundus.** The cervix is located at the same level as the deepest portion of the bladder, and the body and the fundus of the uterus extend craniad from this position. The parallel walls of the vagina extend caudad from the cervix, again in close approximation to the posterior wall of the bladder (Fig. 12–1A).

A small percentage of patients have what is known as a **retroverted uterus.** Normally the body and fundus of the uterus lie against the posterior wall of the bladder in a plane more or less parallel to the sacrum. A retroverted uterus has its fundus tipped dorsally, and its plane is perpendicular to the sacrum. This normal anatomic variant can pose difficulties for the sonographer because the fundus extends so far

posteriorly that gas-bearing bowel may slip between the bladder and uterus, obscuring the view (Figs. 12–1B and 12–2).

The **adnexal regions** lie on either side of the uterus and contain the ovaries, fallopian tubes, and broad ligaments. (The latter are fibrous bands that contain the fallopian tubes and uterine blood vessels and help to support the uterus.) The normal fallopian tubes and vessels are often too small to be seen, but the ovaries are usually visible as small oval structures located somewhere between the uterus and the side walls of the pelvis. The actual location of the ovaries is quite variable. Sometimes they are in close approximation to the fundus or the body of the uterus; on other occasions they may be separated from it by a few centimeters and can even abut the side walls of the pelvis. One ovary may be located craniad, near the top of the uterus, while the other may be deep down by the cervix. Regardless of their location, they are usually easy to identify because they are the only masses normally encountered in the adnexal regions.

The rectum and portions of the sigmoid colon lie dorsal to the uterus and adnexa. This is fortunate, as they usually contain air and cast acoustic shadows. Some ultrasonographers recommend giving the patient a water enema to convert the rectosigmoid colon to a cystic tubular structure and facilitate its identification. While this maneuver can be effective in helping to define the retrouterine structures, it adds complexity and an element of unpleasantness to the procedure. We have found it unnecessary in the majority of scans and reserve it for the occasional instances when we are really confused as to the identity of structures.

Uterine Size and Texture

The average length of the uterus in a premenopausal woman is between 8 and 12 cm.

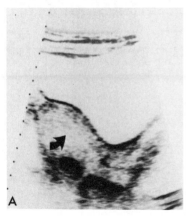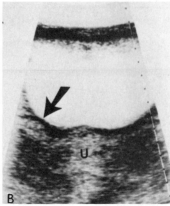

Figure 12–1.   *A.* The uterus is best demonstrated on longitudinal scans. The intensity of the endometrial echoes *(arrow)* varies with the menstrual cycle.
   B. The position of the ovaries is variable, but they can usually be found somewhere between the uterus and the pelvic side walls. This transverse section shows the right ovary *(arrow).* The left ovary was located closer to the cervix. U = uterus.

The width of the fundus is 4 to 5 cm, and of the cervix 2 to 3 cm. In postmenopausal women the uterus is usually about half this size. The uterine echoes are of medium strength, about the same intensity as the liver. The texture of the uterus should be uniform and homogeneous except for the central uterine canal. The intensity of the echoes from the canal varies with the stage of the menstrual cycle. In the first days following a menstrual period, these echoes are of nearly the same intensity as the adjacent myometrium; and the uterine cavity may be difficult to delineate. As the endometrium proliferates in the later phases of the cycle, the echoes become more intense and stand out clearly from the adjacent muscular tissue. Finally, during menstruation the endometrial echoes become quite intense and may contain small focal areas of decreased echo production (Figures 12–1A and 12–3).

Duplication of the uterus is a not uncommon anatomic variation. This condition has a spectrum ranging from complete duplication (two separate uteri and vaginas) to slight broadening of the uterine fundus. It most commonly presents as a widening of the fundus with a small band of myometrium dividing the endometrial echoes into a Y-shaped configuration.

Ovarian Size and Texture

The ovaries vary somewhat in size, but average about 2 to 3 cm in greatest dimension in

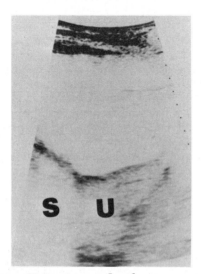

Figure 12–2. A retroflexed, or retroverted, uterus is oriented vertically and is difficult to see clearly. This is a longitudinal midline scan. U = uterus, S = shadow cast by air in colon.

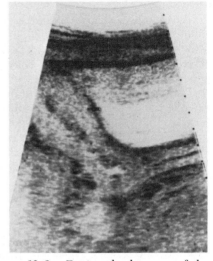

Figure 12–3. During the last part of the menstrual cycle the endometrial echoes become very prominent. Compare this picture with Figure 12–1A, which was obtained during the first part of the cycle.

women during the childbearing years. In both the prepubertal and postmenstrual age groups they may be slightly smaller. The echo intensity of the ovaries is similar to that of the uterus, and they too should have a homogeneous texture. It is common to see at least one small ovarian cyst in menstruating women. These are normal physiologic follicular cysts that arise and regress during the menstrual cycle. Near the time of ovulation, at midcycle, they are usually 1 or 2 cm in diameter but may be as large as 4 cm (Figure 12–4). Following ovulation, the follicular cyst changes to a corpus luteum and may either decrease or increase very slightly in size. When the corpus luteum regresses and menstruation begins, the cystic element rapidly disappears and is no longer visible by ultrasound. The important thing for the ultrasonographer to keep in mind is that these small physiologic cysts are normal findings and do not indicate a pathologic condition.

SCANNING TECHNIQUE

Scanning the pelvis is either duck soup, or it is virtually impossible. When the patient's bladder is full enough to displace small bowel up out of the pelvis, it offers an excellent acoustic window for visualizing the pelvic organs in any scan plane. On the other hand, when the bladder is only partially filled or empty, it can be impossible to make an adequate scan, regardless of how hard the sonographer tries. We cannot emphasize this point enough. For an adequate ultrasound examination of the pelvis to be performed, *the urinary bladder must be full;* attempting a scan with a partially filled bladder is asking for trouble. Not only will you encounter great difficulty in performing the examina-

tion but in all likelihood you will make erroneous diagnoses. You cannot evaluate what you cannot see well.

Practical applications department: It is no exaggeration to say that getting the patient's bladder full is the hardest part of performing a pelvic ultrasound scan. Even though all our patients are instructed to have a full bladder when they arrive for the examination, less than half of them actually do. There are always a variety of excuses, and the sonographer is often made to feel as if the primary goal is torturing the patient. We have found a couple of things that can be useful in this regard. First, the definition of "full" is variable; to many people "full" means only "not empty." As long as they have not just been to the bathroom, they feel that the bladder must be full. For this reason we no longer use the term "full bladder" but rather instruct our patients to drink 32 ounces of fluid one hour before the ultrasound examination and then not to void afterward. It is also helpful if the patient understands why a full bladder is necessary. "We realize that this is uncomfortable for you, and we are not trying to be mean. It is just that we cannot perform an adequate examination unless your bladder is uncomfortably full, and we want to do the best possible job for you."

Determining whether the bladder is adequately distended takes only 10 seconds of scanning. If you can easily find the uterus, you are in business. If only a portion of the uterus is visible, you should immediately stop scanning, take the patient off the table, give her something to drink, and scan another patient while you wait for the bladder to fill. When the bladder is adequately distended, it is easy to see the uterus and adnexal areas in either longitudinal or transverse planes. We routinely use both views.

We begin scanning longitudinally, taking a look at the uterus and then at both right and

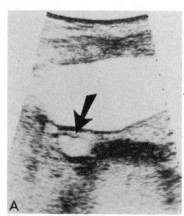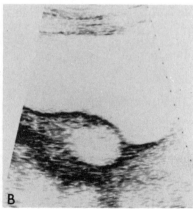

Figure 12–4. Physiologic ovarian cysts are very common and can be large.
A. A follicular cyst *(arrow)* of the right ovary.
B. A corpus luteum cyst of the left ovary in longitudinal section.

left adnexa, including the ovaries. We then change orientation to scan transversely. We start low to see the vaginal walls and sweep craniad through the cervix and the body of the uterus. Each of the adnexa is then examined. Representative views are recorded to document our findings. In normal cases we produce about six hard copies (three longitudinal, three transverse); if there is abnormality, the number of scans recorded will be greater.

PATHOLOGIC APPEARANCE OF THE UTERUS

Size

The size of the uterus alone is rarely an indicator of pathologic change. Uterine size varies slightly during the course of the menstrual cycle, and it shrinks considerably in the postmenopausal state. The most common conditions that cause enlargement of the uterus (besides pregnancy, of course) are **leiomyomata** (fibroids) and **malignant tumors.** While these conditions do cause the uterus to become enlarged, this enlargement is usually focal in nature rather than diffuse.

Texture

As is the case with uterine size, there are very few processes that cause a uniform change in the texture of the uterus, because pathologic conditions that alter the uterine texture almost always do so in a focal manner. The one possible exception to this rule is **endometritis**—inflammation of the endometrium. This process appears as an increased prominence of intensity of the endometrial echoes associated with edema and, consequently, decreased echo production in the adjacent myometrium. These findings are subtle and difficult to recognize, and ultrasound is not a very effective method of making this diagnosis.

Focal Lesions

Focal lesions of the uterus are invariably solid and present as areas of either increased or decreased echogenicity. There are only two basic processes to consider, **leiomyoma** (fibroid) and **malignant tumors** (endometrial carcinoma, cervical carcinoma, and leiomyosarcoma). Un-

fortunately, there is no characteristic difference in the ultrasound appearance of these conditions, and there is no way to differentiate them reliably based on the ultrasound scan alone.

Fibroids are common and are probably a variation of the normal uterine aging process (Fig. 12–5). They are benign tumors of muscle that are seen with increasing frequency with age. Fibroids often undergo degeneration and central necrosis. In the early stage of development they appear as areas of decreased echogenicity in the uterine wall. When degeneration occurs, their echogenicity increases, and they become echo dense. Calcifications with shadowing can be present. Fibroids are sensitive to estrogen levels and may increase dramatically in size during pregnancy.

Endometrial and cervical carcinoma and leiomyosarcoma are much less common than fibroids but ultrasonically have a similar appearance (although calcification is not seen). Unfortunately, there is no ultrasonic pattern that reliably distinguishes these malignant tumors from their benign cousin, and differentiation must be made on the basis of other information such as a Pap smear or endometrial biopsy. The vast majority of focal lesions of the uterus are benign fibroids, particularly in the premenopausal patient. We, therefore, have no hesitation in making this diagnosis whenever we see a focal lesion in the uterus. Even in the older patient with postmenopausal bleeding,

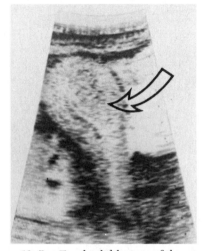

Figure 12–5. Focal solid lesions of the uterus are usually leiomyomas (fibroids). This tumor *(arrow)* has a texture very similar to that of the uterus and is only recognizable because it distorts the endometrial cavity. Many fibroids have high-intensity echoes and some have calcifications that cast shadows.

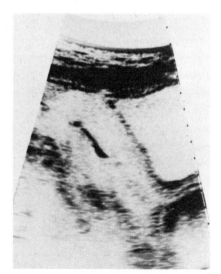

Figure 12–6. An intrauterine device (IUD) produces a loud echo in the endometrial cavity and may cast a faint shadow.

benign fibroids are much more common than malignant tumors.

There is one focal lesion of the uterus that is not really a lesion—the intrauterine contraceptive device, or **IUD**. IUD's are easy to recognize because they produce a very-high-intensity echo that casts a small shadow (Figure 12–6). This echo is normally located within the endometrial cavity; when it arises from the myometrium, it indicates abnormal placement or migration of the device. The usual clinical situation is the missing IUD string. If the characteristic echo pattern cannot be found on good ultrasound scans in these patients, it is strong evidence that the IUD is not within the uterus. (When the IUD lies completely outside the uterus, the device itself may not be recognizable because of bowel gas.) If we cannot find the IUD within the uterus, we like to confirm its absence (or presence outside the uterus) by an x-ray of the pelvis.

PATHOLOGIC APPEARANCE OF THE ADNEXA

First, a word about adnexal disease in general. We find it difficult to make specific pathologic diagnoses in the female pelvis without considerable help from the history and physical findings. Many of the pathologic conditions found here look alike, and it is unusual to encounter any process that has a "typical" or "pathognomonic" appearance. "Why bother

with ultrasound to assess the pelvis, then?" you say. First, we can confirm or exclude the presence of abnormality when physical examination is difficult or equivocal. Second, it is usually possible to localize disease to either the uterus or the adnexa. Finally, *combining* our findings with historical data and the results of physical examination, we can often come to a reasonably specific diagnosis. Although we urge you to be conservative in your statements regarding the findings in pelvic ultrasound examinations, do not become unduly discouraged because you cannot offer specific diagnoses. Most ultrasonologists find themselves in the same boat and must approach the situation in the same way (though many of them will not admit it publicly).

Cystic Lesions

We have already discussed benign **follicular ovarian cysts.** Ovarian cysts less than 3 cm in diameter are virtually always physiologic. Benign conditions that cause cysts larger than 3 cm include **teratomas (dermoids), serous** and **mucinous cystadenomas** of the ovary, **acute** and **chronic infection, endometrioma,** and **ectopic pregnancy** (Figure 12–7). With the exception of mucinous cystadenomas, any of these processes can appear as mixed lesions, which we will discuss in a moment. Unfortunately, it is never

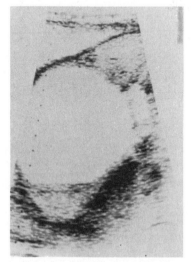

Figure 12–7. Cystic masses in the adnexa can be caused by many conditions such as dermoids (teratoma), cystadenoma, abscess, endometrioma, ectopic pregnancy, and physiologic ovarian cyst. This scan shows a large mucinous cystadenoma.

possible to exclude **malignancy** if a cystic ovarian lesion is found. Age, however, can influence diagnosis; the older the patient, the greater the chance of cancer. For this reason any ovarian cyst of more than 3 cm in a patient older than 30 years of age should be suspected of malignancy.

Ovarian cysts of any type present another problem. They are prone to twist on their pedicles. If this happens, their blood supply may be compromised and the patient will have pain. Therefore, if you encounter an adnexal cyst more than 3 cm in diameter in a patient with pelvic pain, the possibility of **torsion of the cyst** should be considered. (See how the combination of clinical information and ultrasound findings works?)

Solid Masses

Purely solid lesions of the ovary are very uncommon; therefore, if an adnexal mass is completely solid, it is probably *not* of ovarian origin. **Benign** and **malignant ovarian tumors, teratomas,** and **chronic** and **acute pelvic inflammatory disease** will occasionally appear as solid adnexal masses (Figure 12–8). Tumors of the other pelvic organs such as bowel, bladder, and lymph nodes must also be included in the differential diagnosis; but they can almost always be recognized by their location. Finally, **uterine fibroids** may be pedunculated and can, therefore, present as solid adnexal masses rather than as part of the uterus itself.

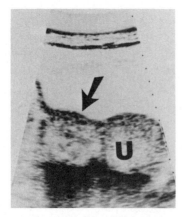

Figure 12–8. Solid adnexal masses are uncommon. They can be caused by benign or malignant tumor, pedunculated uterine fibroid, and chronic abscess. This transverse scan shows a chronic right tubal abscess *(arrow)*. U = uterus.

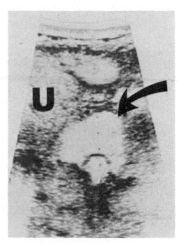

Figure 12–9. Complex adnexal masses are common. The causes include benign and malignant tumors, endometrioma, ectopic pregnancy, and abscess. This mass *(arrow)* was an ovarian dermoid (teratoma). U = uterus.

Mixed Masses

The mixed or complex mass is the most common abnormality of the adnexa. These lesions, which contain both echogenic and echo-free elements, arise from a variety of causes, such as **endometriosis, benign** and **malignant ovarian tumors, teratomas, acute** and **chronic pelvic infection,** and **ectopic pregnancy** (Figure 12–9). Again there is no way to tell these processes apart based only on the ultrasound appearance; the findings on pelvic examination and the clinical setting must be considered if you are to arrive at a specific diagnosis.

ULTRASOUND AND EARLY PREGNANCY

We shall discuss the ultrasound examination during the first 12 weeks of pregnancy (the *first trimester*) in this chapter. This is because the scanning techniques are the same as for the female pelvis and the clinical problems during this period are different from those that arise in the second and third trimesters of pregnancy (which are discussed in the next chapter). There are several questions to be answered during the ultrasound examination.

Fetal Age

First some semantics. It is customary to date gestation from the onset of the mother's last

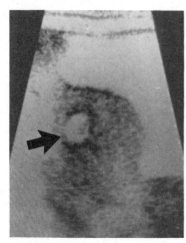

Figure 12–10. The earliest ultrasonic sign of pregnancy is the presence of a small cystic area *(arrow)*—the gestational sac—within the endometrial cavity. This pregnancy is five and a half weeks old (10 days after the missed period).

menstrual period. Because ovulation usually occurs about two weeks later, the fetus is actually two weeks "younger" than the gestational age would suggest. Why, then, use the menstrual period as a reference point? First, women can usually remember when menstrual flow began; and second, ovulation varies; it is not always two weeks after the start of the period. For reproducibility and simplicity the menstrual dating system is useful and is now universally employed.

Fetal age can be determined more accurately in early pregnancy than at any other time. The earliest indication is the appearance of a small cystic area—the **gestational sac**—in the central cavity of the uterus. The sac first appears at about five weeks' gestational age (that is, one week after the first missed period). During the fifth and sixth weeks of gestational age the sac enlarges rapidly but maintains its more or less rounded configuration and contains few discernible internal echoes (Figure 12–10). By the end of the sixth week small echoes from the fetus appear at one edge of the sac; and between the sixth and eighth weeks this collection of echoes rapidly enlarges to assume a lumpy configuration that more clearly represents the developing fetus. Sometime during the seventh or eighth week the pulsations of the fetal heart become visible, and by nine weeks the fetal head should be recognizable and distinct from the fetal body (Figure 12–11). The tenth to twelfth weeks are periods of rapid fetal growth during which head,

body, heart, and limbs become easily discernible.

Because of the rapid change in the fetus during this period, it is usually possible for an experienced ultrasonographer to give a fairly precise estimate of gestational age just by looking at its anatomy; however, most also like to use some sort of objective measurement for the fetal age. In the first trimester, the **crown-rump (C-R) length** has become the most widely accepted method. At this point in fetal development the crown-rump length is defined as the greatest fetal dimension. It is obtained by changing the scan plane until the greatest fetal length is obtained, as shown in Figure 12–11. (There is a reference in the bibliography that gives the relationship between the crown-rump length and the fetal age.)

Short cut department: A pretty good estimation of fetal age in weeks can be obtained by measuring the crown-rump length in centimeters and adding 6.

Toward the end of the first trimester the **biparietal diameter** (BPD) can be determined, and this measurement can be plugged into any of the standard BPD tables to estimate gestational age (see Chapter 13 for more details).

Multiple pregnancy can be recognized early during the first trimester. Count the number of gestational sacs, and you have the number of babies. It is important to look for the fetal pole in all the gestational sacs of a multiple pregnancy in order to establish that each of the fetuses is viable.

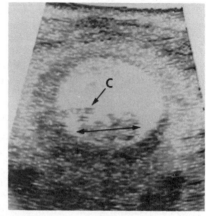

Figure 12–11. From 7 to 12 weeks the crown-rump length *(double-ended arrow)* can be used to estimate fetal age. This fetus is nine weeks old. C = umbilical cord.

Fetal Viability

You will frequently be asked to assess fetal viability, most often in a situation in which the mother is bleeding or the obstetrician cannot obtain a fetal heartbeat by auscultation or Doppler scanning. If the fetus is eight weeks of age or older, a fetal heartbeat should be discernible by ultrasound. An experienced sonographer using a modern real-time scanner can find a heartbeat at that age, and failure to do so indicates fetal death.

If the pregnancy is less than eight weeks of age the detection of a fetal heartbeat may not be reliable (because of resolution limitations of the scanner), and the assessment of fetal viability becomes more difficult. If there is a large discrepancy (that is, more than five weeks) between the expected age of the fetus and its development as seen by ultrasound, fetal death is likely. There is always the possibility, however, that the estimated age of the pregnancy is incorrect, so we prefer to take a conservative approach in these situations. When the development of the fetus suggests a gestational age of less than eight weeks, we do not make a statement as to fetal viability. Instead, we suggest re-examination in 10 days. Normal fetal growth is so rapid during this period that there should be a dramatic change in the overall length and development of the fetus if it is living. Failure of the fetus to increase its crown-rump length or change its anatomic configuration over a 10 day period indicates fetal death.

Who's on first department: There are several somewhat confusing terms used to describe the states of fetal death. **Abortion** is the official medical term to describe all these situations. "Miscarriage" is a lay expression and not a medical one; the corresponding medical term is "spontaneous abortion." An intentional abortion is called "induced" or "therapeutic." Most aborted fetuses are spontaneously passed by the patient; that is, the uterus empties itself of the pregnancy. This is known as a "complete abortion." Sometimes only a portion of the gestation passes, and the remainder is retained within the uterus. This is known as an "incomplete abortion" and is recognizable ultrasonically by the presence of focal areas of increased echoes, possibly with some fluid, in the central uterine cavity. If none of the gestational tissue is passed, the term is "missed abortion." Finally, if a gestational sac is present, but no fetal elements can be seen at a time when they would normally be expected, the condition is termed a "blighted ovum."

Ectopic Pregnancy

Although ultrasound is useful in diagnosing ectopic pregnancy, it cannot stand alone and *must be used in conjunction with the results of a valid pregnancy test.* What constitutes a "valid" pregnancy test? The danger is not so much in a false positive test as in a false negative one, and this means that the test employed must be sensitive enough to pick up only modestly elevated levels of human chorionic gonadotropin (HCG). Ectopic pregnancies seldom progress normally and may not produce levels of HCG as high as normal pregnancies do. If the pregnancy test is one of the drugstore or supermarket do-it-yourself types, it may not be adequate. The current standard (a radioimmunoassay of the "beta sub-unit" of the HCG molecule in maternal serum) is very sensitive. If this widely available test shows normal HCG levels, you can be certain that you are *not* dealing with an ectopic pregnancy, regardless of the ultrasound findings.

If the HCG level is elevated, however, your next objective is to determine whether the pregnancy is located within the uterus. Sometimes the ectopic pregnancy itself can be recognized as a gestation in the adnexal regions, but this is not generally the case (Figure 12–12). The problem is that an ectopic pregnancy does not come to medical attention until it has become symptomatic. This means that the pregnancy has usually been compromised, hemorrhage and disruption of the sac have occurred, it no longer has a typical gestational appearance, and it becomes indistinguishable from many other types of adnexal masses. Sometimes blood can be seen as an echo-free collection in the cul-de-sac behind the cervix. This is an important sign of rupture of an ectopic pregnancy and should never be ignored.

Our criteria for evaluating possible ectopic pregnancy are: (1) The patient must be known to be pregnant by means of a valid pregnancy test. (2) If a gestational sac or pregnancy is seen within the uterine cavity, an ectopic pregnancy can be excluded (twin pregnancies of which one is intrauterine and the other ectopic have been reported but are certainly rarer than hen's teeth). (3) If no gestational sac or fetus is identified in the uterine cavity, an ectopic pregnancy is present. (4) The presence of a mass in the adnexal region is helpful confirmatory evidence of an ectopic pregnancy but is in no way

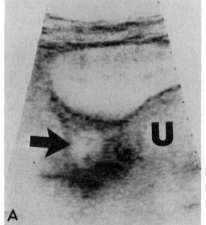
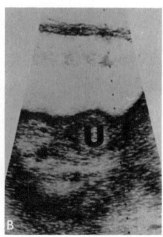

Figure 12–12. There is no characteristic or "typical" appearance for an ectopic pregnancy.

A. This transverse section shows a gestational sac in the right adnexal region *(arrow).* U = uterus.

B. This ectopic pregnancy appears as a complex pelvic mass. U = uterus.

specific. (5) The presence of free fluid in the cul-de-sac behind the cervix is an important sign of intraperitoneal hemorrhage.

Gestational Trophoblastic Disease

The term **gestational trophoblastic disease** refers to a spectrum of diseases characterized by abnormal development of a pregnancy. At one extreme is the benign process of **hydatidiform mole** (molar pregnancy). At the other extreme is the malignant **choriocarcinoma.** Most of these processes are thought to arise from abnormal development of a fertilized ovum.

We like to think of hydatidiform mole as a placenta without a fetus. Its most common ultrasonic appearance is as a large mass of high-intensity echoes that enlarges the uterine cavity. There may be variable amounts of fluid within the mass, but the predominant process is one of high-level echoes indicating solid tissue (Figure 12–13). The total volume of the molar pregnancy is greater than what would be expected for a normal pregnancy of the same age; and, therefore, the uterine size is usually too large for the patient's dates. The molar tissue secretes very high levels of pregnancy hormones (HCG), which cause excessive stimulation of the ovaries and result in the development of large cysts (called **theca lutein cysts**). These cysts are multiple, 2 or 3 cm in diameter, and are often septated; ultrasonically they resemble soap bubbles as seen in Figure 12–13. In fact this appearance is so characteristic that it is usually diagnostic of trophoblastic disease, regardless of the intrauterine findings.

Choriocarcinoma is the malignant form of trophoblastic disease in which the abnormal tissue not only invades the placenta but also metastasizes to distant sites. It is not possible

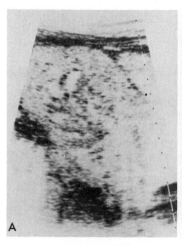
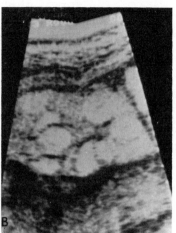

Figure 12–13. Molar pregnancy (gestational trophoblastic disease) has a fairly characteristic presentation.

A. A longitudinal scan through the *uterus* demonstrating high-intensity echoes. There are some cystic areas in the endometrial cavity.

B. A longitudinal section of right *ovary* showing the "soap bubble" appearance of theca lutein cysts.

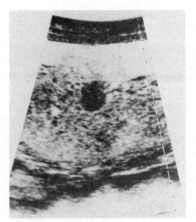

Figure 12–14. Trophoblastic disease can occur in association with a fetus. The high-intensity echoes in this placenta were areas of trophoblastic disease. The fetus is usually abnormal in such cases.

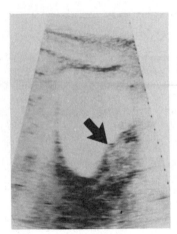

Figure 12–15. The normal prostate (*arrow*) is located in the midline beneath the *caudad* portion of the bladder as seen on this longitudinal scan.

to differentiate benign from malignant trophoblastic disease on the basis of the ultrasound appearance, because both produce the same high-intensity echoes in the intrauterine cavity as well as ovarian stimulation.

Trophoblastic disease can coexist with a normal pregnancy, either as a twin gestation or in a mixed gestation. In these situations, however, it is unusual for the normal part of the pregnancy to carry to term. In cases of mixed gestation, the fetus is usually abnormal and has three sets of chromosomes (triploidy) and multiple somatic developmental defects. This rare situation can be suggested when a large placenta with focal areas of increased echoes is seen early in pregnancy (Figure 12–14).

Male Pelvis

PROSTATE SIZE AND TEXTURE

We will mention briefly the possibilities of using ultrasound in the male pelvis. The most obvious object of interest is the prostate, which is located in the midline, adjacent to the posterior surface of the bladder. Whereas the uterus extends from the most dependent portion of the bladder craniad, the prostate runs from the most dependent portion of the bladder caudad (Figure 12–15). The normal prostate is about 3 cm in diameter and round in configuration. Its echo texture is mid level, approxi-

mately the same as the liver or the uterus, and normally the gland is homogeneous. The prostate causes a slight indentation on the posterior wall of the bladder, but this is not prominent unless it is enlarged.

PATHOLOGIC APPEARANCE OF THE PROSTATE

Only two things go wrong with the prostate: it enlarges—**benign prostatic hypertrophy**—and it develops **cancer.** Both of these processes have the same ultrasonic appearance. As the prostate gets larger, it produces a more prominent indentation on the floor of the bladder and often projects quite prominently into its lumen (Figure 12–16). There is loss of the normal echo texture, and focal areas of increased echogenicity are seen. There has been little interest in scanning the prostate at our institution; and although there are some laboratories that perform this examination routinely, the definitive role of ultrasound in prostatic evaluation remains to be elucidated.

Urinary Bladder

Finally, we must not forget to look at the urinary bladder. Ultrasound is not a widely used procedure for problems that arise in this organ, but it certainly is possible to see tumors, particularly those that project from the wall,

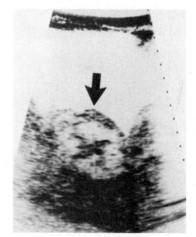

Figure 12–16. Benign prostatic hypertrophy and carcinoma both cause the gland to enlarge and its echo texture to become heterogeneous. This patient has benign hypertrophy *(arrow)*. Transverse section.

and in some instances wall thickening due to cystitis has been noted. It is worthwhile to spend a few seconds examining the bladder to look for such lesions. The more common abnormalities such as simple cystitis and muscular hypertrophy do not have a characteristic ultrasound appearance and usually cannot be recognized.

BIBLIOGRAPHY

Hall, D. A., Mann, L. E., Ferrucci, J. T., Jr., et al.: Sonographic morphology of the normal menstrual cycle. *Radiology 133*:185 (1979).
(A good review of the changes in the uterus during normal menstruation; this article is an "atlas" of the "normal" appearance of the uterus.)

Requord, C. K., Wicks, J. D., and Mettler, F. A., Jr.: Ultrasonography in the staging of endometrial adenocarcinoma. *Radiology 140*:781 (1981).
(This article discusses the problems in separating benign and malignant uterine disease by using only the ultrasound scan.)

Walsh, J. W., Taylor, K. J. W., Nasson, J. F. M., et al.: Gray-scale ultrasound in 204 proved gynecologic masses. *Radiology 130*:391 (1979).
(A good discussion of the spectrum of pelvic disease. We have not found the "specific sign" for dermoid reliable, however.)

Brown, T. W., Filly, R. A., Laing, F. C., et al.: Analysis of ultrasonic criteria in the evaluation for ectopic pregnancy. *American Journal of Roentgenology 131*:967 (1978).
(This is a good discussion of the ultrasonic findings in ectopic pregnancy. Unfortunately, beta sub-unit pregnancy tests were not widely available in these patients and, therefore, the overall diagnostic accuracy is less than we expect nowadays.)

Boricelli, L., Orsini, L. F., Rizzo, N., et al.: Estimation of fetal age during the first trimester by real time measurement of fetal crown-rump length and biparietal diameter. *Journal of Clinical Ultrasound 9*:71 (1981).
(A thorough discussion of a variety of measurements for predicting fetal age. This article has tables of crown-rump length and BPD as well as a nomogram that uses both.)

Munyer, T. P., Callen, P. W., Filly, R. A., et al.: Further observations on the sonographic spectrum of gestational trophoblastic disease. *Journal of Clinical Ultrasound 9*:349 (1981).
(The best available discussion of this group of diseases.)

Chapter 13

PREGNANCY

Pregnancy is big business, and for the ultrasonographer the pregnant uterus is a steady source of interesting challenges—the staff of life of the general ultrasound lab. It has been estimated that currently one out of every five pregnancies in the United States is studied by ultrasound. Many enthusiasts are predicting that within 10 years' time virtually every fetus will be observed in utero and that previously lethal intrauterine mishaps will be recognized and successfully treated. Even if these predictions are overly optimistic, there is no question that ultrasound will play an increasingly important role in prenatal care. Moreover, most obstetrical ultrasound examinations are fun: The patients are young and healthy, the studies reasonably easy to perform, and the results exciting to both the parents and the examiner. In the preceding chapter we covered the first trimester: the diagnosis of early pregnancy, problems with abortion and fetal viability, and ectopic and trophoblastic gestations. In this chapter we shall concentrate on the developing fetus from 10 weeks to maturity or "term."

SCANNING TECHNIQUES

The organ-oriented examination is just as appropriate for use in pregnancy as in general scanning. We are searching for several kinds of information, which should be obtained in logical order. In addition to the fetus itself we want to study the two organs directly involved in the pregnancy—the uterus and the placenta. To conduct the examination in an expeditious manner and to be certain of reliable results, we believe you should examine each organ or clinical problem in a predetermined sequence, resolving each issue before moving on to the next. You must be flexible in selecting scan planes when performing an obstetrical examination. The uterus and the placenta do not move; but the fetus is active, and locating a scan plane that provides the information you

are seeking requires a sharp eye and a quick hand. In general the entire lower abdomen is available as an acoustic window because the enlarged uterus displaces the air-filled bowel. *It is still important to insist on a distended urinary bladder so as to be able to get a good look at the cervix and the lower uterine segment; the quality of your study will be compromised unless the acoustic window of the bladder is there to help you.*

The limited field of view of real-time scanners is something of a handicap in examining pregnancies because there is no way to include the whole uterus from fundus to cervix on a single scan. At first this drove us crazy. We had been used to the global views produced by the manual or articulated arm scanners, and we despaired of ever being able to manage with the postage stamp glimpses that the real-time machine gave us. We developed a systematic approach to the problem, a variation of the organ-oriented exam, however, and before long we had reassured ourselves that the loss of the large field of view was more than compensated for by the increased flexibility and clearer definition that the real-time instrument offered.

To begin, we get our bearings by scanning *longitudinally* over the lower uterine segment in the midline to see the cervix, the upper vaginal walls, and the urinary bladder. We continue, still longitudinally in the lower uterine segment, by scanning to the right and left of midline. The scanner is then moved upward toward the uterine fundus. From this we have more or less gotten the lay of the land and have made representative hard copies to record what we have seen. We are now ready to go after our two main intrauterine objectives, the fetus and the placenta. Our evaluation is designed to count the number of fetuses, determine their position (or presentation), estimate fetal age (and size), and assess fetal well-being. (Each of these areas is discussed in detail in the following sections; however, to show how the organ-oriented obstetrical examination is conducted, we will touch briefly on each here.)

So far in our look at the uterus we have restricted ourselves to scanning longitudinally. Because babies are generally not oriented strictly either longitudinally or transversely, the scan plane will now have to be altered in order to get the best look at the fetus. The scanner is moved about until the fetal head is seen, and once it is located, views of the head for biparietal diameter (BPD) measurements are made. At the same time the ultrasonographer assesses the intracranial anatomy so that any abnormality there can be recorded. Next, the fetal trunk—including the heartbeat, the abdominal organs, and the spine—is evaluated. This may require considerable adjustment of scan plane by the operator; but by the time it is completed there should be no question about fetal position and the general status of the baby. Now we look at the placenta. Its lowest extension toward the cervix is recorded longitudinally; then it is examined transversely, and scans are made to show its farthest extension to both right and left sides of the uterus. With this overview of the obstetrical exam behind us, we are now ready to look more closely at its various components.

FETAL PRESENTATION

Fetal presentation (or "lie") is a term that refers to the position of the baby relative to the cervix and is important information for the referring obstetrician. There are three basic lies: cephalic, breech, and transverse.

Cephalic presentation is the most common. In this lie the fetus is oriented head down and bottom up. Nature organized childbirth for cephalic lies. The fetal head is an efficient dilator of the cervix and the birth canal and helps speed normal vaginal delivery. Also, the fetal head is the largest part of the baby; therefore, if there is cephalopelvic disproportion (that is, if the fetus is too large to pass through the maternal pelvis), it will become apparent early in the course of labor before the fetus has progressed so far as to get stuck. Cephalic presentation is easily diagnosed by a longitudinal scan at the cervix: If the fetal head is seen on this view, the lie is cephalic (Figure 13–1).

Breech presentation is the opposite of cephalic: The baby is head up and bottom down. Unfortunately, breech presentation makes labor and delivery more difficult. The buttocks are not as effective as the head in dilating the cervix and vagina; and because they are smaller than the head, when there is cephalopelvic dispro-

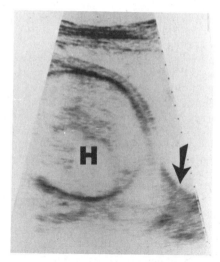

Figure 13–1. Cephalic presentation is the most common fetal orientation. This midline sagittal scan shows the head (H) abutting the cervix (*arrow*).

portion, the fetus can progress a long way down the birth canal before discovering that it cannot get out. Most severe fetal injuries during childbirth occur with breech presentations. A breech presentation can also be identified in the midline scan at the cervix. If, instead of seeing the fetal head in this section, there is the fetal abdomen or buttocks, then it is a breech (Figure 13–2). To be certain of the diagnosis, the scan plane should be moved up along the midline to the top of the uterus to demonstrate that the fetal head is in the fundus.

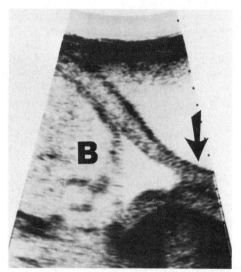

Figure 13–2. In breech presentation the buttocks (B) are next to the cervix (*arrow*) on a midline sagittal scan.

In a **transverse presentation** the fetus is lying sideways with its head on one side of the uterus and its bottom on the other. The fetus will either be "back up" (the back is toward the fundus of the uterus and the limbs toward the cervix) or "back down" (the back toward the cervix and the limbs toward the fundus). Many obstetricians like to know whether a transverse lie is back up or back down, so that when a cesarian section is performed, the uterine incision can be made to avoid the fetal trunk. Transverse lie should be expected when the head is not seen in the midline longitudinal plane, either in the cervical region or in the fundus.

Remember that the fetus is mobile and fetal presentation changes many times during the course of pregnancy. Prior to 28 weeks it is unusual for the fetus to have a stable position, and the designation of fetal lie is not very useful during this period. After 28 weeks, however, changes in fetal position are much less common, and the knowledge of the fetal lie becomes important to the obstetrician.

NUMBER OF FETUSES

In general the diagnosis of multiple pregnancy is not difficult; one has only to count the number of fetal heads.

Easier said than done department: During early pregnancy when fetuses are active, it can sometimes be difficult to prove that there are actually two fetuses instead of a single very active one. Here is another case where real-time makes all the difference in the ease of examination.

Usually in twin pregnancy one fetus will be cephalic and the other breech. When both babies have the same lie, the diagnosis is more difficult because the second fetal head is often obscured in the shadow cast by the first. It is most important to vary the scan planes to avoid the problem of missing twin pregnancy. Multiple gestations greater in number than twins are infrequent. They present a great challenge to the ultrasonographer faced with the problem of trying to figure out which heart goes with which head and who is lying on top of whom. When more than three fetuses are present, it may be impossible to sort the whole affair out; these examinations take great patience and more than a little imagination.

In multiple gestations it is useful to attempt to decide whether there are one or two placentas. Sometimes it is impossible to tell, but if you are clearly able to see two separate placentas, you know that you are dealing with non-identical twins. Regardless of whether twins are identical or not, each will always have its own separate amniotic cavity, so you should expect to be able to identify a membrane separating the twins.

Stating the obvious department: Finding twins doubles the ultrasonographer's work. There are now two fetuses to be examined for age and well-being; and the ultrasound report must specify which data go with which fetus.

THE PLACENTA

Placental localization is also of major importance to the obstetrician. Before the advent of ultrasound there was no safe, reliable method of obtaining this information. Normally the placenta lies near the fundus of the uterus or on one of the side walls, well above the internal cervical os. In a small percentage of cases, however, it is located low in the uterus; and if a portion of it extends over the cervical os, it is known as a **placenta previa.** Placenta previa not only makes vaginal delivery impossible (by blocking the outlet of the uterus), it can also be dangerous for the mother because, near term, when the cervix starts to dilate for delivery, the blood vessels of the placenta may be torn and life-threatening hemorrhage may result. Bleeding can be provoked either by the onset of labor itself or by a pelvic examination during this critical period.

Minor bleeding *not* associated with placenta previa is common in normal pregnancies, but when bleeding occurs near term, the obstetrician must always assume the presence of placenta previa until it has been disproved. In the past this usually meant the patient had to be hospitalized, and before a pelvic examination could be performed an emergency operating room had to be prepared in case massive hemorrhage occurred. Only a small number of mothers with third trimester bleeding actually had placenta previa, so the rigmarole of setting up operating rooms and so forth caused a great deal of unnecessary trouble and expense. Ultrasound has changed all this; we can now clearly see where the placenta is located and should be able to diagnose placenta previa easily and quickly with nearly 100 per cent accuracy.

The placenta can generally be recognized

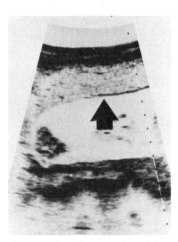

Figure 13–3. The placenta has a homogeneous echo texture slightly more intense than the uterine wall. Its internal surface is covered by a smooth lining, the chorionic plate *(arrow)*.

from the fourteenth week of pregnancy on. It is a chunky, fusiform organ applied to one of the uterine walls. Its normal echo pattern is monotonously homogeneous, and the strength of the echoes within it is always greater than in the adjacent uterus. The internal surface of the placenta is covered by a smooth lining, the chorionic plate, which appears on the ultrasound scan as a well-defined, strong, continuous line (Figure 13–3). There is often a layer of decreased echoes between the placenta and the underlying wall of the uterus, which we will discuss in a moment.

A placenta located on the anterior or side walls of the uterus or in the uterine fundus is easy to visualize. When the placenta lies on the posterior wall of the uterus, however, things can be more difficult because the fetal bones cast shadows that obscure things. All is not lost, however, because you can assume that if the placenta is nowhere else in the uterus, it must by default be on the posterior wall, hidden in the shadows of the fetus. Another clue to the posterior placenta is that the fetus seems to float more toward the anterior wall of the uterus, displaced away from the back wall by the "unseen" placenta. In the end of course, you will feel more confident if you can see the placenta directly, and here the real-time scanner comes to your aid. The fetal parts that obscure the placenta move, and continued observation will provide occasional glimpses of the placenta on the posterior wall, so you can be sure of its position.

As we have mentioned, when a tongue of placenta reaches down near the cervix, the

diagnosis of placenta previa must be entertained. There has been a great deal written about making this diagnosis, and in the past ultrasonographers have been prone to overdiagnose previas. There are several reasons for this. Sometimes it is difficult to see the actual location of the internal cervical os because it may be obscured by the fetal head or hidden under the symphysis pubis. Also, an overdistended urinary bladder can squeeze the lower portion of the uterus and make the internal os appear to be higher than it actually is. In this instance a low-lying placenta may appear to extend over the os as a placenta previa. This error can be avoided by rescanning the patient after she has emptied her bladder. Once the pressure from the urinary bladder has been removed, the lower uterine segment will distend, and you will be able to see that the placenta does not extend to the internal os.

When evaluating the lower uterine segment for the presence of the placenta, we recommend that you scan in longitudinal section just above the symphysis pubis and move the scan plane back and forth from side to side. The cervix should be readily identifiable. Next look on the uterine walls above, below, and on either side of the cervix to see if there is any placenta in this region. If no placenta is seen, previa can be excluded absolutely. If the placenta is present here and it crosses the cervical os, attaching to *both the anterior and the posterior uterine walls*, the diagnosis of previa is certain (Figure 13–4). If the placenta extends down near

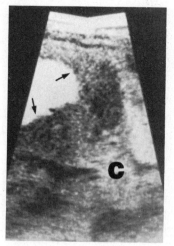

Figure 13–4. Placenta previa can be difficult to diagnose on sagittal scans. The chorionic plate must curve around the cervix and it must attach to both the anterior and posterior walls of the uterus *(arrows)*. C = cervix.

the cervix, but you are unsure whether it actually crosses it, switch the scan plane around to transverse and scan at a level somewhat above the cervix. Be careful to angle the plane of the scan so that you cut across the uterus more or less perpendicularly to its long axis. Now, maintaining this angle, move the scan plane down toward the cervix and observe what happens to the placenta and the amniotic fluid. If the placenta occupies the whole central portion of the uterus before the cervix is reached, there is a placenta previa. We call this the "bull's eye" sign, because that is what the picture resembles (Figure 13–5). If amniotic fluid appears and you cannot make a bull's eye picture in transverse section, you are not dealing with a placenta previa. Finally, in light of what we said about the full urinary bladder, all potential placenta previas should be examined both before and after emptying the bladder. A true placenta previa will be present on a post-void scan as well as on a pre-void study.

Go west young man department: There is a commonly observed ultrasound phenomenon known as **placental migration.** This term describes the observation that during the course of pregnancy placentas seem to "migrate" toward the uterine fundus. A patient examined during early pregnancy may often appear to have a low-lying placenta or a placenta previa, yet this same patient examined at 33 weeks will show a placenta far away from the cervix. Does the placenta really wander? Many authorities think not. Instead, they feel that the uterus enlarges predominantly in the lower segments, and as pregnancy progresses the lower portions of the uterus "grow" away from the placenta. Other obstetricians feel that indeed the placenta may migrate. They point out that the vascularity of the lower uterus is much poorer than that of the fundus and suggest that portions of the placenta that are implanted near the cervix may atrophy during the course of pregnancy because of poor blood supply, while the remainder of the placenta grows toward the well-nourished fundus. Whatever the explanation, the observation of "placental migration" is valid. Many times what appears to be a placenta previa at 25 weeks will be gone near term; therefore, the ultrasonologist should always recommend a repeat examination near term in any case of suspected placenta previa.

Although the placenta is easily seen after 14 weeks, it is sometimes difficult to identify reliably during earlier stages of pregnancy. The placental echoes are always of higher intensity than those in the wall of the uterus, and during early gestation it can generally be assumed that the wall of the uterine cavity that has the highest-intensity echoes will be the placental site. For reasons that we cannot explain it is sometimes difficult to be certain of placental location in pregnancies as advanced as 15 weeks. We have been embarrassed more than once by a placenta that appeared to change from posterior wall at 15 weeks to anterior wall at 24 weeks. (Maybe the placenta really does migrate.) At any rate we urge you to be cautious when diagnosing placental localization before 15 weeks of gestational age and not to be

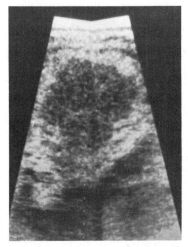

Figure 13–5. Placenta previa gives a "bull's eye" appearance on transverse scans through the lower uterus. The high-intensity central portion of the bull's eye is the placenta; the less intense rim is the uterine wall.

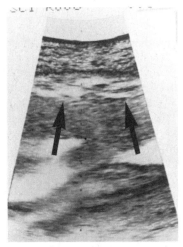

Figure 13–6. Occasionally a sonolucent area is present between the placenta and uterine wall. This is a normal variant and probably represents blood lakes or sinusoids.

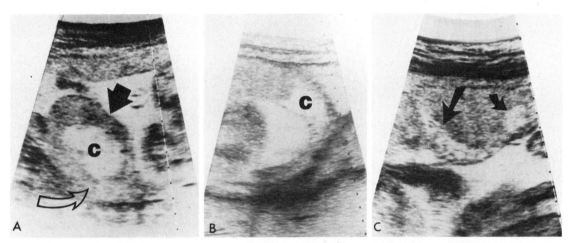

Figure 13–7. Abruptio placenta, while common, is not often recognized by ultrasound.
A. A large blood clot (c) separates the placenta *(short arrow)* and uterine wall *(curved arrow).*
B. The edge of the placenta is rounded and separated from the uterine wall by an echo-free blood clot (c).
C. There is a deep cleft in this placenta, running from the chorionic plate down to the base *(straight arrow).* The curved arrow points to a focal echo-poor area. These are intraplacental hematomas.

surprised if it is not where you expect it when you re-examine the patient later.

Even though during most of pregnancy the placenta has a uniform echo texture of higher intensity than the adjacent uterine wall, there may be a band of very low-intensity echoes between the placenta and the myometrium. Most ultrasonologists believe this band represents a vascular area of blood lakes and sinusoids beneath the placenta (Figure 13–6). This echo-free zone can mislead the inexperienced and cause confusion with a condition known as premature separation of the placenta, or **abruptio placentae**, a frequent cause of bleeding in pregnancy. Most often premature placental separations are of little consequence; the pregnancy is not disturbed, and the only manifestation is a placental scar seen after delivery has occurred. In spite of the fact that it is presumed that abruption is the cause for most bleeding during pregnancy, the diagnosis is relatively infrequently made by ultrasound. There are three signs of separation of the placenta that will confirm the diagnosis if they are present: (1) large echo-free spaces beneath the placenta, which represent retroplacental clot; (2) echo-free areas that extend deep into the placenta from the chorionic plate (also probably blood clot); and (3) thickening of the placenta, especially if associated with rounding of its edge (Figure 13–7).

During early pregnancy the placental texture is uniform. As pregnancy progresses, however, focal heterogeneity appears within it. These areas may be echo-free or regions in which the echoes are of high intensity, or a combination of the two (Figure 13–8). Such changes are generally more common toward the end of pregnancy; in fact at one time it was thought that this appearance was a reliable sign that the fetus was mature. Unfortunately, this concept has not been borne out by experience, and one cannot rely upon the observation of placenta heterogeneity as an indicator that the fetus is

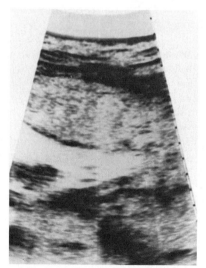

Figure 13–8. The texture of the placenta becomes more heterogeneous as the pregnancy nears term. Placental heterogeneity is not a reliable sign of fetal maturity, however.

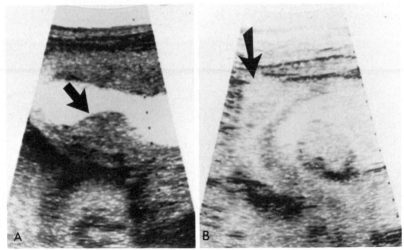

Figure 13-9. A mass in the wall of the uterus is either a fibroid or a focal contraction.

A. This focal contraction has exactly the same echo texture as the adjacent uterine wall. Focal contractions are common in the first 20 weeks of pregnancy and may persist for 30 minutes.

B. A fibroid usually has a different echo texture than the adjacent uterine wall. In this case the texture was nearly the same, however, and the diagnosis was made by showing that the mass was present over a two-day period.

mature enough to survive extrauterine existence without difficulty.

Before leaving the topic of the placenta, we must not forget the uterine wall itself. Normally the myometrium is relatively echo-free and uniformly thinned around the amniotic cavity; however, focal areas of uterine wall thickening are common. When these are seen, there are two diagnoses to consider: **leiomyoma** (fibroid) and **local contraction.** Leiomyomas contain echoes either higher or lower in intensity than the adjacent myometrium, while contractions have the same echo texture as the adjacent uterine wall. Fibroids will not vary in size or shape, but contractions will often disappear over a period of several minutes. When you encounter a focal mass in the uterine wall, go on to study other things. Then come back to the mass at the end of the examination. If it is still present and has not changed and if its echoes are not of the same intensity as the rest of the uterine wall, you are more likely dealing with a fibroid than with contraction (Figure 13-9).

FETAL AGE

Perhaps the most important, and certainly the most frequently requested, information to be obtained from an obstetrical examination by ultrasound is a determination of the fetal age.

Virtually all assessments of fetal abnormality are based on an estimation of fetal age, and the reliability of this estimation influences greatly the appropriateness of all subsequent clinical decisions. As an example, consider a woman who presents in labor. Is this normal labor in a mature pregnancy, or is it premature? It all depends on the age of the fetus. If the fetus is at term, the onset of labor is normal. On the other hand, if the fetus is only 32 weeks of age, labor is premature and, unless terminated, could result in the delivery of a premature infant. Estimating fetal age has always been, and continues to be, a difficult problem.

First, what is a normal gestational term, that is, how many weeks is it normal for the fetus to remain in the uterus before the onset of spontaneous labor and delivery? The generally accepted time is 39 or 40 weeks. (All pregnancies are measured in weeks and counting begins at the first day of the last normal menstrual period. Thus, according to this system, by the time the mother misses her first period, she is already four weeks pregnant.) Like all things in life there is an expected variation in the "normal" length of pregnancy. If a large number of normal pregnancies are followed, it turns out that delivery occurs somewhere between 37 and 43 weeks; and if delivery dates are put on a graph, they form a bell-shaped curve. The curve begins at 37 weeks and tapers off at about 43 weeks, a six-week spread. The peak of the curve is at 39 weeks and three days, and this serves as the basis for the statement that a "normal" pregnancy lasts between 39 and 40 weeks. We can see that, all other problems aside, it is difficult to be precise about how long the baby should be in the mother, because we do not know if the pregnancy was predestined to be a 37 week or a 43 week gestation.

A second complication arises from difficulties in identifying the onset of the last menstrual period. One would think that this date would be easy to determine, but in a sizable percentage of pregnancies, it is not known reliably. There are many reasons for this, such as irregularity of periods, uncertainty as to what is a normal period and what may be bleeding associated with early pregnancy, and pregnancy occurring without a previous period in a patient who has recently stopped birth control pills.

Third, fetuses grow at different rates, and the size of the uterus is not a reliable indicator of the age of the baby. Pregnancies with breech presentations usually appear larger than those with cephalic presentations. Twins will obviously take up more room and require a larger uterus than single pregnancies. The amount of amniotic fluid and general body structure of the mother will alter the carrying angle and height of the uterus.

Ultrasound allows us to look at the fetus *in utero* and has provided a way of getting more accurate estimations of fetal maturity. The basis of the ultrasound determination of fetal age beyond the first trimester is the **biparietal diameter** or **BPD**. In the very early days of clinical ultrasound, it was observed that the

fetal head tended to grow at a uniform rate regardless of what was happening to the rest of the fetus. Moreover, it was observed that most fetal heads seemed to grow at roughly the same rate, which was independent of the size of the parents, their ethnic origin, or general health. Large series of patients were examined in many localities throughout the world, and tables relating the fetal head size to gestational age were constructed. These tables provide the foundation for ultrasonic dating of pregnancy.

Before we can use such tables, we must know how to obtain a BPD measurement. This is actually a simple process; all we do is make a picture of the greatest transverse diameter of the fetal head (Figure 13–10). When a real-time scanner is used, this is no trick at all; it is even fairly easy with articulated arm machines. There are three rules for making acceptable pictures of the head for measurement of the BPD. (1) The head must be symmetrical and either round or elliptical in shape. (2) If a midline echo is present, it must be located in the midline and not to one side or the other. (3) At least four or five pictures must be obtained, each in a slightly different scan orientation; the measurements on these pictures should differ by no more than 2 mm.

When these three criteria are met, the greatest transverse diameter of the skull (the BPD) can be easily determined. There is confusion in the literature about where the measurements should be taken. The line that makes up the image of the fetal head on the scan can vary considerably in width, and it is possible to measure from three different places on this line:

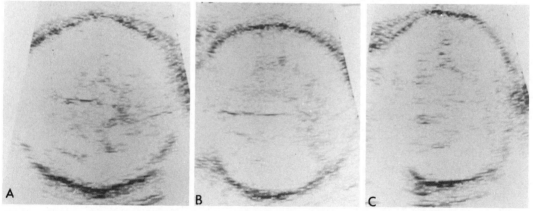

Figure 13–10. We do not believe it is useful to have a precise orientation for measuring a biparietal diameter. All three of these scans would be satisfactory even though the orientation is different in each. The only criteria for a satisfactory scan are that the diameter be the greatest obtainable, the skull surfaces be symmetrical, and the midline echo, if present, be in the midline.

(1) the leading edge (also designated as the outer surface of the fetal calvarium nearer the transducer and the inner wall of the far side), (2) the trailing edge (the inner wall of the near surface and the outer wall of the far side), and (3) a point midway between these two. In the end it makes little difference which you select, because errors introduced by different measurements are tiny and do not affect the overall accuracy of the BPD age estimation process. We think it is easiest and most reproducible to make the measurements from the midpoint of the skull surface echoes. Using this technique will give you measurements less likely to be adversely influenced by a faulty gain setting that produces wider than optimum lines.

Oversimplification Department: Some authors, particularly in Europe, are extremely fastidious in their criteria for obtaining BPD images and would shudder

at our rather cavalier approach to this process. While we have no objection to precision and do not wish to foster sloppy work, it is important to bear in mind that the whole BPD business is imprecise at best because we are dealing with a biologic population in which there is great variation. Obtaining a more refined measurement will not greatly increase the accuracy of the final result. *Consistency* is important, however, and it is imperative that you develop good technique in examining the fetal head so that your results are reproducible.

Once you have obtained the BPD, simply look up the estimated fetal age on one of the widely available charts. Table 13–1 is ours. It was derived from European data, but it is similar to many other charts derived in various parts of the United States, Western Europe, and Japan. Notice that it contains both an average and an age range. Just as the length of the "normal" pregnancy varies, so the rate of

TABLE 13–1. Biparietal Diameter Chart

BPD (cm)	MEDIAN (wks)	RANGE (wks)	BPD (cm)	MEDIAN (wks)	RANGE (wks)
2.5	12½	11 –13½	6.3	25	23½-27
2.6	13	11½–14	6.4	25½	24 –27
2.7	13½	12 –14	6.5	26	24 –27½
2.8	13½	12½–14½	6.6	26	24½–28
2.9	14	12½–15	6.7	26½	25 –28½
3.0	14	13 –15½	6.8	27	25 –28½
3.1	14½	13 –15½	6.9	27	25½–29
3.2	15	13½–16	7.0	27½	26 –29½
3.3	15	14 –16½	7.1	28	26 –29½
3.4	15½	14 –16½	7.2	28	26½–30
3.5	16	14½–17	7.3	28½	26½–30½
3.6	16	15 –17½	7.4	29	27 –31
3.7	16½	15 –18	7.5	29	27½–31½
3.8	16½	15½–18	7.6	29½	28 –32
3.9	17	16 –18½	7.7	30	28 –32½
4.0	17½	16 –19	7.8	30½	28½–33
4.1	17½	16½–19	7.9	31	29 –33½
4.2	18	17 –19½	8.0	31	29 –34
4.3	18½	17 –20	8.1	32	29½–34½
4.4	19	17½–20	8.2	32	30 –35
4.5	19	17½–20½	8.3	32½	30 –35½
4.6	19½	18 –21	8.4	33	31 –36
4.7	20	18½–21½	8.5	34	31½–36½
4.8	20	19 –21½	8.6	34½	32 –37
4.9	20½	19 –22	8.7	35	32½–37½
5.0	20½	19½–22	8.8	35½	33 –38½
5.1	21	19½–22½	8.9	36½	33½–39
5.2	21½	20 –23	9.0	37	34 –40
5.3	21½	20½–23½	9.1	37½	34½–41
5.4	22	20½–24	9.2	38	35 –42
5.5	22	21 –24	9.3	39	36 –>42
5.6	22½	21½–24½	9.4	39½	36½–>42
5.7	23	21½–25	9.5	40	37 –>42
5.8	23	22 –25	9.6	41	37½–>42
5.9	23½	22 –25½	9.7	42	38 –>42
6.0	24	22½–26	9.8	>42	38½–>42
6.1	24½	23 –26	9.9	>42	40 –>42
6.2	24½	23 –26½	10.0	>42	41 –>42

growth of the "normal" fetal head varies. If we obtained BPD measurements on 1,000 normal babies who were 28 weeks of age, we would find that we had a bell-shaped curve that had a peak at 7.1 cm but ranged from 6.6 to 7.7 cm. The BPD table is designed to show this variation. Thus, a single BPD measurement of, say, 7.4 cm tells us that the fetus could be anywhere from 27 to 31 weeks of age, but its most likely age is 29 weeks. (For those of you who like statistics, the age range in this table is from the tenth to the ninetieth percentile).

Biparietal diameter measurements have added considerable objectivity to the estimation of fetal age, but they still leave something to be desired from the clinical standpoint. Notice that in early pregnancy the age range is small and the dating is fairly precise; during the later stages of pregnancy, however, from 30 weeks onward, the age range is nearly six weeks. Obviously, a single BPD measurement late in pregnancy is not of much value. To reduce this variation, then, it is important that fetal age be determined as early as possible, ideally before the twenty-fifth week. This is especially important whenever the need for gestational dating can be foreseen (a "high-risk" pregnancy).

Spot Quiz: Not infrequently, a patient will have two ultrasound examinations, one in early pregnancy and the other near term. The BPD measurements from these examinations may give different estimations of fetal age. In this situation, which measurement is more likely to be correct? Answer: the date obtained at the earlier examination should be the more accurate (see Table 13–1).

Several methods of improving the accuracy of fetal age estimation have been developed. None has been universally accepted by obstetricians, but we will briefly discuss two of the more popular ones.

The first of these entails the measurement of the circumference of the fetal skull. The key to accuracy here is making certain that one obtains a picture of the skull showing the greatest circumference possible. This means that the plane chosen must not only have the longest biparietal diameter, but also the greatest anteroposterior dimension. The flexibility of the real-time scanners makes choosing the correct plane relatively easy. First, scan until you can place the midline echo of the falx in the middle of the skull. Maintaining that degree of inclination, move the plane up and down through the fetal head until you get the greatest BPD. Then vary your angle slightly and locate the longest AP diameter. The picture you obtain

will almost always include the strong echoes of the falx as well as the two short paramidline echoes of the walls of the cavum septi pellucidi anteriorly. If your scanner is not equipped with an electronic means of measuring the circumference, this measurement can be obtained from the hard copy by using an inexpensive map mileage calculator and an appropriate conversion scale. Head circumference correlates well with gestational age (there is a reference in the bibliography that will provide you with a graph for relating gestational age to circumference), but this determination is time consuming, and we use it only when it appears that the fetal head is unusual in shape and the BPD is more likely to produce an incorrect age.

Another popular method for refining gestational age is known as the Growth Adjusted Sonographic Age, a concept introduced by Sabbagha. The theroretical foundation of the method seems sound. We know that there is a normal variation in the rate of fetal head growth; some babies grow rapidly, while others grow more slowly. The simple BPD charts assume that every fetus is growing on the average line. If it were possible to determine whether the fetus is a rapid grower or a slow grower, it would be possible to use a BPD chart that more accurately reflects this growth rate and hence would have less variability in the final age estimation. In order to determine the growth rate of the fetus, it is necessary to have two BPD measurements separated by 8 to 10 weeks. This means the patient must be examined first at about 20 to 22 weeks' gestation and then again near 30. The BPD obtained at the second exam is compared with the expected BPD for that length of gestation. Then adjustment of the fetal age can be made according to whether the baby appears to be growing rapidly or more slowly. Using these two measurements, it is claimed, gives an age estimate that is accurate to within two weeks. Further details of this method are available in the references in the bibliography.

In the final analysis, however, when it is known that precise estimation of fetal age will be important in managing the patient, the easiest way to guarantee accuracy is to examine the fetus early. The error and variation then are much less, and the gestational age can be reliably determined with a single examination.

FETAL WELL-BEING

Modern scanners now enable the ultrasonographer to conduct an effective examination of the fetus. Many gross anatomic defects affecting the baby have been recognized and reported. A comprehensive review of such defects is beyond the scope of this text; a survey of the fetus should, however, be a part of every obstetrical examination and with a bit of standardization can be easily performed. We will review the technique of the examination and leave details of specific fetal abnormalities to the references in the bibliography.

Because the fetal head is the most easily recognized part of fetal anatomy, it is always best to begin there. The plane of the scan should be adjusted until the fetal skull is seen axially, that is, in the same plane as the standard computed tomograph (if you imagine that you are looking down on the skull from above, you have the correct orientation). Landmarks within the head allow us to recognize the posterior and the anterior ends of the skull. The most important of these is an arrowhead configuration produced by the cerebral peduncles as they pass through the tentorium of the cerebellum (Figure 13–11A). The scan plane at this point is low in the skull, and the "arrow" points toward the occiput (the posterior end of the skull). As the level of the plane of the scan is moved toward the vertex (or top of the skull), two short parallel lines that are separated by several millimeters of echo-free space will appear ante-

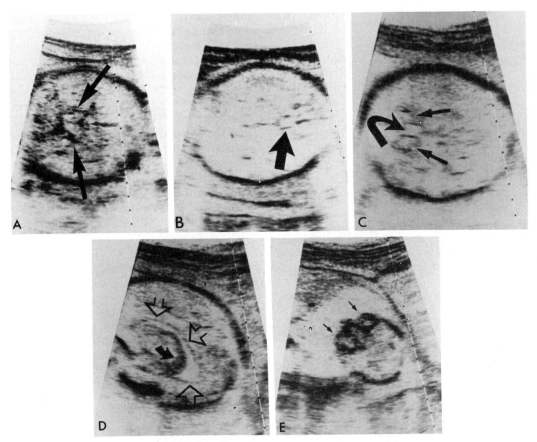

Figure 13–11. Modern scanners demonstrate much fetal intracranial anatomy.

A. Near the base of the skull the cerebral peduncles produce an easily recognized "arrowhead" which points toward the occiput *(arrows)*. A similar picture may be produced by the tentorium.

B. The cavum septi pellucidi is readily recognized as two short lines separated by an echo-free space.

C. It is difficult to identify the lateral ventricles. Beyond the first half of the second trimester they can be seen *reliably* only when dilated. This fetus has hydrocephalus, and the frontal horns of the dilated lateral ventricles *(straight arrows)* are seen adjacent to the cavum septi pellucidi *(curved arrow).*

D. If the lumen of the lateral ventricle can be *definitely* identified, the fetus has hydrocephalus. This diagnosis is most easily made on sagittal sections of the fetal head. Open arrows = lateral ventricle, solid arrow = choroid plexus.

E. Scans through the base of the fetal skull show the orbits *(arrows)* and nose.

riorly (Figure 13–11B). While there is some controversy about this, most people now believe that this echo-free space is produced by the cavum septi pellucidi. (Many ultrasonologists recommend using the level in which the walls of the cavum are visible to measure the BPD. We believe this is fine as long as this level also produces the greatest BPD).

Identification of the lateral ventricles is not reliable unless they are dilated. Some ultrasonographers feel that the outer walls of the lateral ventricles can be recognized as lines running parallel to the midline echo. This has not been our experience, and we have had particularly poor results when trying to predict hydrocephalus by measuring the distance of these lines from the midline echo. We are not certain that this structure does in fact represent the lateral wall of the body of the lateral ventricle; furthermore, we have not been able to diagnose hydrocephalus on the basis of the relationship of ventricular to hemispheric width as demonstrated on axial scans of the fetal head alone. Artifacts can create echo-free areas that simulate big ventricles and mislead the unwary. As pregnancy progresses, the ventricles occupy relatively less of the intracranial space, and dilated ventricles become more easily discernible. The danger exists primarily in a false positive diagnosis of hydrocephalus in the 18–22 week range.

By the time the third trimester begins the *lumen* of the normal lateral ventricle is less than 1 mm wide and should not be seen. If the ventricular lumen is visible then, the fetus is hydrocephalic (Figure 13–11C and D). On the other hand, if the lumen is not visible (with a scanner that can resolve the cavum), the fetus is not hydrocephalic, regardless of any measurements of "lateral ventricle lines."

Other parts of the skull can be identified. Figure 13–11E shows a scan through the base of the skull. The orbits and the petrous portions of the temporal bones, separating middle and posterior fossas of the skull, are recognizable. It is important to be able to use these simple landmarks for orientation; they make deviations from normal much easier to identify and interpret.

After looking at the skull, the remainder of the fetus is examined from head to pelvis by moving the level of the scan plane while keeping it more or less perpendicular to the long axis of the fetal spine. We usually make several passes up and down the baby's trunk to take in everything; again, an organ-oriented approach

is useful. (Not every aspect of the fetus can be evaluated with equal facility throughout pregnancy; for example, the vertebrae can be seen rather well between 16 and 20 weeks; however, after that the fetal spine is apt to be flexed, and this limits our ability to assess it. On the other hand the visceral organs of the fetus are seen with increasing facility as they enlarge during the second and third trimesters).

We begin by looking at the vertebral column, from the cervical spine to the pelvis (Figure 13–12). Next we look at the heart (and perhaps count the fetal pulse), the upper abdomen (liver, stomach, and kidneys), and the urinary bladder. It is important to perform this fetal survey on every patient in order to develop a feel for what is normal; then when you are requested to examine a baby for a specific abnormality, you will know what to expect.

The fetal heartbeat is always easily visible in the second and third trimesters. Absence of heartbeat is the sine qua non for making the diagnosis of fetal death, and with the quality of the image available on contemporary scanners, we have no hesitancy in making that diagnosis if heart motion is not seen in the thorax.

The stomach can be seen because the baby swallows amniotic fluid and the filled stomach produces an echo-free structure in the left upper quadrant of the abdomen. The liver is also easily recognizable, and after about 18 to 20 weeks we can generally trace the umbilical vein into the liver to its junction with the left branch of the portal vein. When we wish to measure the circumference of the abdomen, the plane perpendicular to the fetal spine at the level

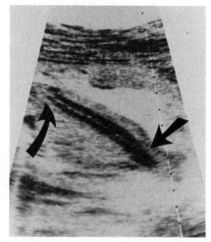

Figure 13–12. The fetal spine should be examined from the neck (*curved arrow*) to the sacrum (*straight arrow*).

where the umbilical and the portal veins join is the one we select for hard copy and measurement (Figure 13–13).

Further down in the fetal abdomen we see the kidneys lying alongside the spine. Occasionally in normal babies the pelvicalyceal systems can be seen because they are slightly distended; but any time the collecting systems and ureters are seen as echo-free structures, one has to be suspicious of an anomaly of the fetal urinary tract producing obstruction. Observation of the fetal urinary bladder is of paramount importance because it provides the best evidence of the presence of functioning renal tissue.

Finally, the fetal limbs also can always be seen with real-time scanners, and the bones identified. A substantial body of literature is being built up reporting observations of long bones and other aspects of limb development in various pathologic states as well as in normal fetuses. In the future it will probably be worthwhile for the ultrasonographer to be accustomed to sorting out the fetal limbs, and we urge you to practice this in your routine scanning.

Adequate evaluation of the fetus depends upon our being able to identify the various fetal parts, and the volume of amniotic fluid is an important factor in this. If there is enough fluid so that the limbs are free to move away from the body and there is fluid between the fetal

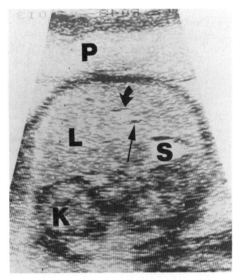

Figure 13–13. The fetal abdomen should be measured on a scan perpendicular to the fetal spine at the level of the junction of the umbilical vein *(short curved arrow)* and the left portal vein *(straight arrow)*. L = fetal liver, S = fetal stomach, K = fetal right kidney, P = placenta.

trunk and the walls of the uterus, we can generally do a good job of looking at the baby. On the other hand, if the volume of amniotic fluid is small, we will be in trouble. In such instances your expectations for satisfactory assessment of the fetus will have to be lowered.

AMNIOTIC FLUID VOLUME

The volume of amniotic fluid can be an important clue to the presence of a serious problem with pregnancy. Because polyhydramnios (too much fluid) and oligohydramnios (too little fluid) are conditions that may bode ill for the fetus, we want to be able to tell the referring physician if either exists. With experience you will develop a feel for the range of normal so that you can recognize when there is too much or too little amniotic fluid (more about the signs later). If you are using a static scanner, it is possible to estimate the volume of the uterus (and indirectly the amniotic fluid) by calculating the total intrauterine volume (TIUV); however, if you do this, you will soon realize that there is a wide variation in normal, and the TIUV often falls into the "gray zone," not clearly abnormal in either direction. (If you use a real-time scanner, the relatively small field of view makes it impossible to estimate the TIUV.) We, therefore, rely upon experience; that is, we "eyeball it" and decide when the amniotic fluid volume is abnormal. We have found that we have been just as accurate with this method as with any of the more "scientific" measurements.

Recognition of **oligohydramnios** is not difficult because the fetal anatomy is obscured. There is not enough fluid for the limbs to float away from the body, and the fetus usually lies against the placenta or the uterine wall. If you are having trouble recognizing the various parts of the fetus, think oligohydramnios. Before 23 weeks **fetal renal disease** is the usual cause of oligohydramnios. Fetal urine contributes significantly to amniotic fluid volume; therefore, when urine volume falls or is absent, amniotic fluid volume is reduced. Later in pregnancy **premature rupture of membranes** and **fetal growth retardation** (IUGR) must also be considered.

Polyhydramnios usually does not develop until the third trimester and may be difficult to recognize in its early stages. The findings are the opposite of those seen in oligohydramnios; that is, the fetus is displaced unusually far from the uterine wall and the fetal trunk and limbs are very easily seen. When the fetus is lost in a giant fishbowl of fluid, think polyhydramnios.

Most cases of polyhydramnios are not associated with any recognizable abnormality, and the increased fluid does not appear to affect the outcome of the pregnancy adversely. Of pathologic cases of polyhydramnios, approximately half are associated with an abnormality of the fetus and the other half are due to maternal difficulties. The cause of polyhydramnios is uncertain; it has been postulated that reduced fetal swallowing, increased loss of fluid because of defects in the fetal skin, and placental insufficiency are contributing factors.

The most common fetal anomalies associated with polyhydramnios involve the central nervous system, and **neural tube defects** such as **anencephaly, encephalocele,** and **meningomyelocele** are the most prevalent. Gastrointestinal anomalies make up the second largest group, and here the lesion almost always involves an obstruction such as **duodenal** or **jejunal atresia. Hydrops fetalis** and **fetal cardiac anomalies** are less common causes.

Maternal problems that lead to polyhydramnios include **diabetes mellitus, pre-eclampsia, congestive heart failure,** and **infection.** Most of these also produce the syndrome of hydrops fetalis (polyhydramnios, fetal edema and ascites, and thickened placenta), but there is rarely anything specific about the uterine ultrasound findings that will enable you to make a definitive diagnosis.

FETAL WEIGHT

Obstetricians like to have an estimate of the fetal weight. There is an obstetrical condition known as **intrauterine growth retardation,** or **IUGR,** in which the fetus seems to develop poorly in the uterus and is subject to increased risk of perinatal death and complications. A fetus has intrauterine growth retardation if its weight is lower than expected for the gestational age. (How much lower is controversial, and every obstetrician will have his own "standard"). Tables of expected fetal weights for various gestational ages are available, so what is needed to identify IUGR is some way of estimating the fetal weight in utero.

In the mid 1970's the total intrauterine volume, or TIUV, obtained popularity for diagnosing this disorder. The TIUV was an estimation of the total volume of the uterus; in severe growth retardation this total volume was decreased. The problem with the TIUV measurement was that it was insensitive and indirect; and because of their restricted field of view. TIUV cannot be determined with most real-time instruments. We no longer employ this measurement.

It seems more logical to us to estimate fetal weight and relate this to gestational age in order to identify the fetus whose growth is retarded. Empirical formulas have been developed to predict the fetal weight on the basis of a series of measurements obtained by ultrasound. The formulas differ from institution to institution; we like the one developed at Yale, which is described in the bibliography. The advantage of this method is that it is fairly accurate and requires only two measurements, the biparietal diameter and the abdominal circumference, both of which are easily obtained.

Cold water department: We, personally, have encountered considerable frustration in diagnosing IUGR because the whole problem is complex and poorly understood clinically—there is neither any widely used definition of the condition nor any universally accepted treatment. The reference by Deter in the bibliography goes into the problems in some detail.

AMNIOCENTESIS

In most high-risk pregnancies amniocentesis will be performed to help evaluate fetal well-being. Ultrasound has proved to be almost indispensable in guiding this procedure because it enables the operator to avoid passing the needle into the placenta or the fetus. The techniques for ultrasound-guided aspiration or biopsy have been described in many previous publications (see bibliography). We do want to point out, however, that it is important that the patient not be moved after the amniocentesis site has been selected by ultrasound. The fetus may change position rapidly, and what was an acceptable puncture site while the patient was on the scanning table may be inappropriate if the patient leaves and goes to a different location for the amniocentesis. Also, it is always advisable to rescan immediately following amniocentesis to verify that the fetal heart rate has not changed. We have not found it necessary to use any of the special transducers developed for aspiration biopsy nor to monitor the entrance of the needle into the amniotic cavity.

PERSPECTIVE

Before leaving this chapter we would like to suggest a reporting format for obstetrical examinations. We not dictate a report in most obstetrical cases, but have developed a preprinted, "fill in the blanks" report that fits easily into the patient's chart (Figure 13–14). This type of report has several advantages. (1) It is standardized so that the same information always appears in the same location regardless of which individual is reporting the ultrasound scan. (2)

The form can be filled out quickly by the ultrasonologist and requires no typing, proofreading, or other delays associated with secretarial duties. It is ready to go as soon as the patient leaves the ultrasound scanning room. (3) Because all the important items must be filled in, it provides a built-in check on the adequacy of the examination.

As you can see, obstetrical ultrasound is a big area, and we have only given you an overview in this chapter. We have stressed the well-accepted "bread-and butter" uses of ultrasound

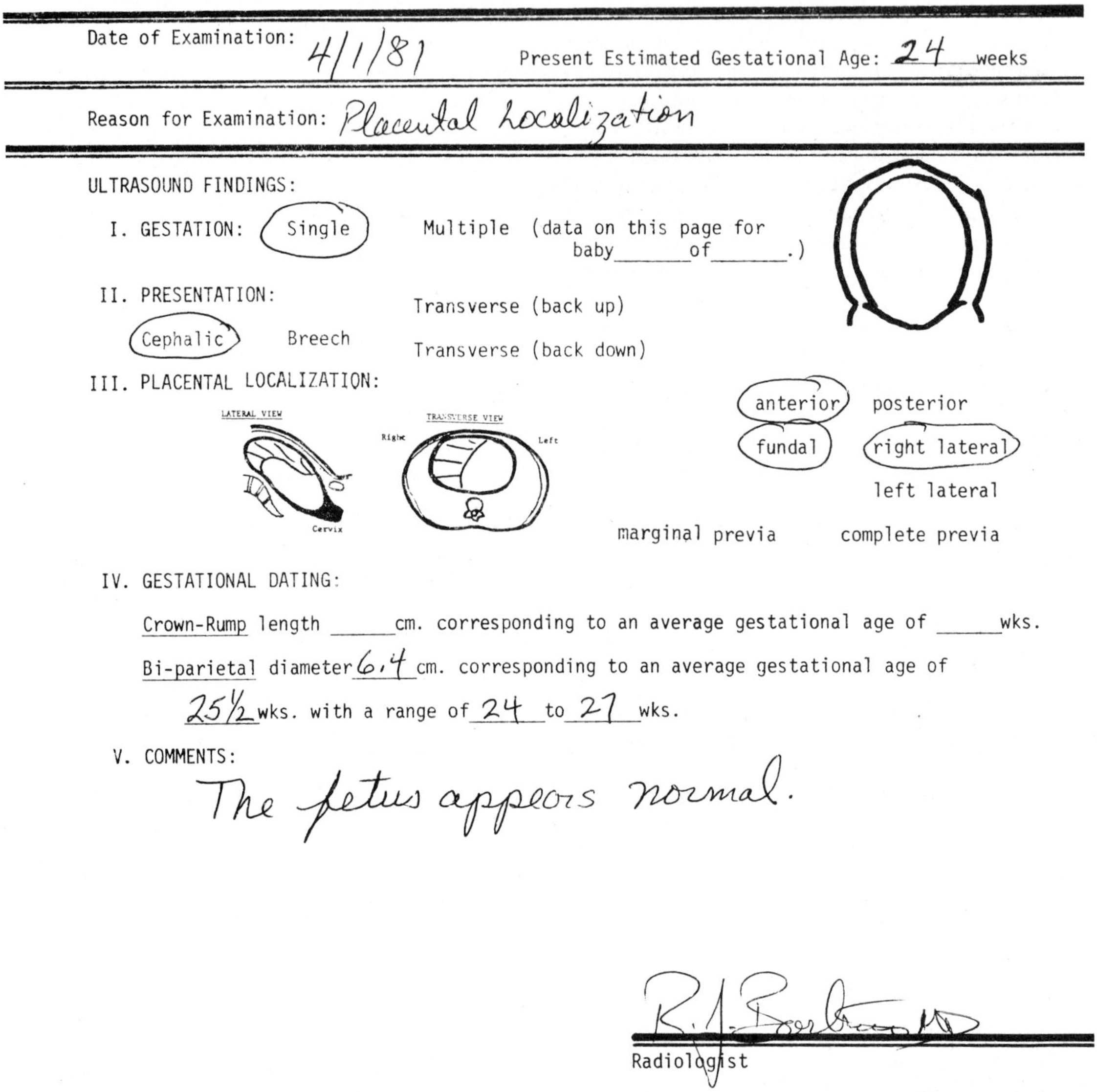

Date of Examination: 4/1/81   Present Estimated Gestational Age: 24 weeks

Reason for Examination: Placental Localization

ULTRASOUND FINDINGS:

I. GESTATION: (Single)   Multiple (data on this page for baby_____ of _____.)

II. PRESENTATION:
(Cephalic)   Breech
Transverse (back up)
Transverse (back down)

III. PLACENTAL LOCALIZATION:

LATERAL VIEW   TRANSVERSE VIEW   Right   Left   Cervix

(anterior)   posterior
(fundal)   (right lateral)
left lateral
marginal previa   complete previa

IV. GESTATIONAL DATING:

Crown-Rump length _____ cm. corresponding to an average gestational age of _____ wks.

Bi-parietal diameter 6.4 cm. corresponding to an average gestational age of 25½ wks. with a range of 24 to 27 wks.

V. COMMENTS:
The fetus appears normal.

Radiologist

Figure 13–14. We use a preprinted, "fill-in-the-blanks" report form for obstetrical examinations: The "comments" section is for discussing fetal well-being. Our report is designed to provide the information *our* clinicians want from the study; you should design your report form to provide the information *your* clinicians desire.

in obstetrics to help you get started. There are many other things you can measure, look at, and do; but unless you have special interests, we suggest that you confine your observations to a few simple and reproducible findings. You should learn to recognize the fetal lie and placental position easily and become comfortable with making or excluding the diagnosis of placenta previa. You should be able to get five or six pictures for BPD measurement in a few minutes, regardless of how unusual the fetal position. The appearance of the fetal anatomy should become second nature, so that gross anatomic disorders are immediately apparent. When you can do all these things well, you will be able to provide useful scans for referring clinicians. After you have established a diagnostic base, you will find yourself experimenting with some of the more esoteric and less well-established uses of ultrasound scanning.

BIBLIOGRAPHY

Hobbins, J. C., ed.: *Diagnostic Ultrasound in Obstetrics.* Churchill Livingston, New York, 1979.
(This is an excellent short monograph on obstetrical ultrasound.)

Sabbagha, R. E. *Ultrasound in High-Risk Obstetrics.* Lea & Febiger, Philadelphia, 1979.
(An even shorter monograph that deals mainly with the concept of growth-adjusted age. Most of this material is also covered in the book cited above.)

Chiun, D. M., Filly, R. A., and Callen, P. V.: Predictions of intrauterine growth retardation by total intrauterine volume. *Journal of Clinical Ultrasound* 9:175 (1981).
(The authors share our opinion that TIUV is of limited value.)

Shepard, M. J., Richards, V. A., Berkowitz, R. L., et al.: An evaluation of two equations for predicting fetal weight by ultrasound. *American Journal of Obstetrics and Gynecology* 142:47 (1982).
(This is the method we use to estimate fetal weight and IUGR. Don't be scared off by the title; the computer has printed out a table, and all you need to do is plug in a BPD and abdominal circumference and look up the fetal weight.)

Deter, R. L., Harrist, R. B., Hadlock, F. P., et al.: The use of ultrasound in the detection of intrauterine growth retardation: a review. *Journal of Clinical Ultrasound* 10: 9 (1982).
(An excellent review of this nebulous problem. This is required reading for anyone who deals with IUGR.)

Mishkin, M., Balm, R. S., Allen, L. C., et al.: Ultrasonic assessment of the fetal spine. *Radiology* 132:131 (1979).
(There are countless case reports of various fetal anomalies scattered in the literature. Here is one on the most common clinical question you are likely to be asked.)

Bartrum, R. J., Jr., and Crow, H. C.: *Gray-Scale Ultrasound.* First edition. W. B. Saunders Co., Philadelphia, 1977, Chapter 13.
(If you are not familiar with the technique of ultrasonically guided puncture or biopsy, this is an illustrated lesson on how to do it.)

Hobbins, J. C., Grannum, P. A. T., Berkowitz, R. L., et al.: Ultrasound in the diagnosis of congenital anomalies. *American Journal of Obstetrics and Gynecology* 134:331 (1979).
(A concise, but relatively complete, review of the spectrum of congenital anomalies that you might encounter in obstetrical ultrasound.)

Filly, R. A., Golbus, M. S., Carey, J. C., et al.: Short-limbed dwarfism: ultrasonographic diagnosis by mensuration of fetal femoral lengths. *Radiology* 138:653 (1981).
(Here is a paper representative of the increasing interest in the evaluation of fetal limbs.)

Alexander, E. S., Spitz, H. B., and Clark, R. A.: Sonography of polyhydramnios. *American Journal of Roentgenology* 138:343 (1982).
(A nice pictorial essay that reviews the mechanisms and the etiologies of polyhydramnios: all you will need to know presented concisely and clearly.)

Chapter 14

SCROTUM

The development of the high-resolution, limited-range (a.k.a. "small parts") scanner has opened new vistas for ultrasound imaging. These instruments, which utilize special pulse length circuitry and high-frequency transducers, provide axial resolution on the order of 1 mm over a limited range (about 5 cm). They are also real-time; that is, the scanning movement is automated so that visualizing small structures that are difficult to immobilize is not a problem. For structures or organs small enough for the limited range (for example, the scrotum, thyroid, carotid artery, and some very small neonatal brains) the ultrasound scans can be truly striking. The results in the scrotum are a case in point. Not only can we visualize small details of the scrotal contents, but we can even make precise pathologic diagnoses as well. Here is an area where ultrasound is a dramatic and valuable addition to the diagnostic process.

NORMAL APPEARANCE

Anatomy

Figure 14–1 is a diagrammatic representation of the scrotum and its contents. The testicle itself is elliptical (shaped like a rugby ball) and occupies most of the scrotum. It is composed of multiple sperm-producing cells and tubules (seminiferous ducts), all of which drain toward one side where they converge and exit into the epididymis. The epididymis is a tubular structure that lies along one margin of the testicle and extends over its entire length. In the epididymis the sperm-containing ducts continue to merge until they join into a single duct—the vas deferens—which runs in the spermatic cord from the testicle into the pelvis. Besides containing the vas deferens, the spermatic cord also carries the arteries, veins, and lymphatics that supply the testicle. Like the seminiferous ducts, these vessels also branch and divide in the epididymis to enter the testicle itself.

The scrotal sac and its contents—the testicle, epididymis, and spermatic cord—are all invested with a smooth lining membrane called the tunica. This membrane is analogous to the peritoneum that lines the abdominal cavity and covers its contents. The portion of the membrane that lines the scrotum itself is called the tunica vaginalis, while the portion that covers the testicle and spermatic cord is called the tunica albuginea. There is a small amount of fluid within the tunica that serves to lubricate the surfaces and allows the testicle and spermatic cord to move and slide freely.

Size

The average testicle is about 4 cm in length by 3 cm in diameter. The much smaller epididymis is dumbbell-shaped with focal enlargements at each extremity—the globus major and the globus minor. The globus major and the globus minor can be up to 5 mm in diameter, but the portion of the epididymis that connects these two is very thin, usually only 1 mm or so in thickness.

The small amount of fluid between the layers of the tunica is most easily seen near the poles of the testicle, where the thickness of the fluid may measure 3 or 4 mm.

Texture

The testicle produces high-intensity echoes that are completely uniform—the most homogeneous organ that we examine with ultrasound. As we shall see, any deviations from homogeneity are abnormal. The epididymis has an echo texture nearly identical with that of the testicle and, therefore, is difficult to separate from the testicle itself. Sometimes the globus major and minor can be recognized by their slightly bulbous shapes. Fortunately, pathologic conditions of the epididymis decrease its echogenicity and make it easier to visualize. If you

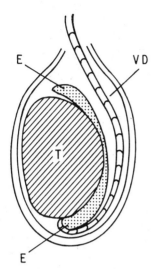

Figure 14–1. The testicle, epididymis, and vas deferens are the intrascrotal organs. T = testicle, E = epididymis, VD = vas deferens.

have difficulty separating the epididymis from the testicle, it means that the epididymis is normal. The spermatic cord contains both solid fibrous tissue and blood vessels and is very heterogeneous. Normally the diameter of the lumens of the blood vessels and vas deferens is just at the threshold of resolution of the scanner, and identification of these individual structures in the cord is not possible. Figure 14–2 shows a normal scrotum.

SCANNING TECHNIQUE

Scanning with one of the limited-range scanners is simple because the organs or areas to be scanned are small and superficially located, and there is little interference by gas and bone.

Usually all that is required is to place the transducer over the area of interest and move it back and forth from side to side so that all portions of the organ are investigated. The scrotum actually presents the most difficulty because its contents are very movable; therefore a system for immobilization must be devised. After considerable trial and error, we have learned to ask the patient to move his thighs together; then we place a towel underneath the scrotum to support it further. Each testicle must be examined individually. This is done by stabilizing the testicle with one hand (gently, of course!) while we move the scanner with the other hand, first longitudinally, then transversely. The transducer cannot actually be moved along the surface of the scrotum, but must be placed in one spot and angled. After all possible angles in one position have been scanned, the transducer is lifted off the skin and replaced a centimeter or two to one side and the process is repeated. The mechanics of this procedure are not as complicated as they sound, and you will get the hang of it quite quickly. The only thing to keep in mind is that a thorough examination must be made, and this usually requires many different transducer positions. With many of the small parts scanners it is not possible to visualize the entire length of a normal testicle because of the limited field of view. This means, of course, that the sonographer has to be careful to move the scanner so as to cover each testicle completely. As always, be sure to record representative hard copy views, at least three longitudinal and three transverse; more if an abnormality is encountered.

Elitist department: We believe that, in general, the quality of the ultrasound equipment is secondary to the skill and persistence of the operator when it

Figure 14–2. A. The normal testicle produces high-intensity homogeneous echoes. (The scale markers are spaced at 2.5 mm for all the illustrations in this chapter.)
B. The globus major of the epididymis (*curved arrow*) is difficult to distinguish from the adjacent testicle (*straight arrow*).

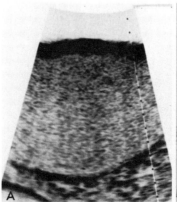
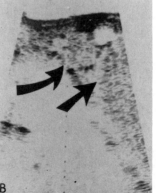

comes to getting information from an ultrasound scan; but in scrotal scanning, this is probably not true. Because of the mobility of the testicle, it is difficult to make satisfactory scans with a static scanner, and real-time instruments have proved to be not only easier to use but capable of producing superior scans. The resolution and detail of conventional abdominal scanners is too poor to see the fine anatomy that enables one to make the highly specific diagnoses we shall describe. We do not mean to say that you should not be scanning the scrotum if all you have is a conventional scanner, but you should not expect the results that are possible with one of the dedicated high-resolution units.

PATHOLOGIC APPEARANCE

Size

Enlargement or shrinkage of the testicle is uncommon. Generalized enlargement of the testicle can be seen with **acute inflammation (orchitis)**. In this case the internal texture of the testicle is usually heterogeneous with ill-defined, permeative areas of decreased echogenicity (Figure 14–3). The clinical setting is usually characteristic: The testicle is excruciatingly tender, so much so that the patient will probably not allow an ultrasound examination.

Acute ischemia (torsion) of the testicle can also cause generalized enlargement but, in our limited experience, does not alter the echo texture. With ultrasound alone it is usually not possible to be certain of the diagnosis, but again the clinical presentation is fairly typical: testicular pain with enlargement and homogeneous echo texture.

Cold water department: Some authors are enthusiastic about using Doppler ultrasound to detect blood flow, or its absence, in the scrotum. Although our experience is limited, we have not found this helpful, and in one case of complete testicular torsion and ischemia the Doppler pulsations were identical to those on the uninvolved side.

Generalized shrinkage of the testicle has been described in cases of completed **testicular infarction** and **atrophy** from either ischemia or orchitis (especially mumps orchitis). In both situations the echo pattern may be normal, but in many cases of infarction there are often areas of decreased and increased echogenicity. On occasion there will be shadowing behind high-intensity echoes indicating focal areas of calcifications.

Excessive Fluid in Tunica

Probably the most common pathologic condition of the scrotum is a **hydrocele**. This is the presence of excess fluid within the tunica and is easily recognized by either clinical examination or ultrasound. Figure 14–4 is an example of hydrocele; it is easy to recognize the excessive fluid surrounding and outlining the testicle. The hydrocele itself is not considered a significant lesion, but it may be associated with other abnormalities of the testicle, especially malignant tumors. Therefore it is important to examine the testicle carefully whenever a hydrocele is identified. Examination is mandatory if a hydrocele develops suddenly or if it changes size.

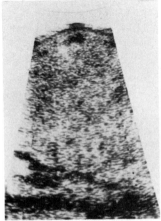

Figure 14–3. Acute testicular inflammation (orchitis) enlarges the testicle and decreases the homogeneity of its texture.

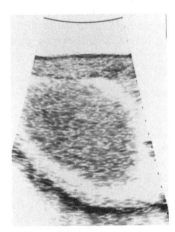

Figure 14–4. The testicle is surrounded by fluid when a hydrocele is present.

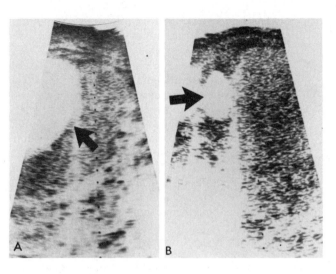

A

B

Figure 14–5. Spermatoceles can be large or small and can arise in either the testicle or the spermatic cord.

   A. A large, intratesticular spermatocele.

   B. A small spermatocele of the epididymis.

Focal Cystic Mass

Figure 14–5 shows two different focal cystic masses in the scrotum; one is in the spermatic cord and the other within the testicle. Regardless of location, focal cystic masses in the scrotum are virtually always benign. They are particularly common in the epididymis and cord. When they contain sperm, they are properly termed **spermatoceles.** (Of course, as ultrasonologists, we cannot see sperm, so we cannot be more specific in our diagnosis than "cyst of the epididymis or testis or cord.") The cause and significance of spermatoceles is not completely understood; the important thing is that they are all benign and generally of no concern.

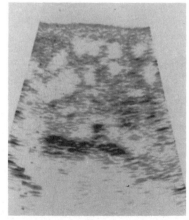

Figure 14–6. Varicoceles are a tangle of veins in the scrotum.

Multiple Cystic Masses

We have never encountered multiple cystic masses within the testicle itself; multiple cysts are always located in the epididymis, the spermatic cord, or the tunica. The vast majority of these masses are **varicoceles**—nests of small, dilated veins (Figure 14–6). Some varicoceles are small, and the venous channels measure only a millimeter or so in diameter; these are frequently referred to as **microangiomas.** When the venous channels are 3 mm in diameter or larger, the term *varicocele* is commonly used. As with spermatoceles, the etiology and importance of varicoceles is not well understood. Because many urologists feel that they can be associated with tumors of the testicle, the testicles should be carefully examined when a varicocele is identified.

Figure 14–7 shows multiple cystic areas occupying the entire tunica space and enlarging it. Actually the cystic spaces are the normal areas, and it is the septa between them that are abnormal. This appearance is seen in the recovery phase of either scrotal **inflammations** or **hemorrhage** or a combination of both. During the acute phase of these processes, the space within the tunica is filled with either pus or blood; as the process resolves, the inflammation or blood clots are liquefied and resorbed, leaving an underlying honeycomb network of fibrous tissue known as synechiae. As healing progresses further, even this underlying reticulum will disappear, and eventually the scrotum will return to a more normal appearance. The

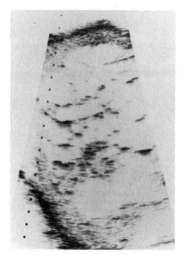

Figure 14–7. Scrotal synechiae are secondary to infection or hemorrhage.

testicle in these situations is usually normal in appearance unless it has been injured by the primary disease process.

Focal Solid Mass

The testicle is normally composed of high-intensity echoes with a very homogeneous pattern. Whenever there is an area where the echoes vary in intensity, it is always abnormal and worrisome. Most focal masses appear as areas of decreased echo production, but occasionally there may also be some high-intensity echoes. A focal solid lesion must be considered

carcinoma until proved otherwise. Sometimes the tumor is large, but even small 5 mm masses must be further evaluated (Figure 14–8).

There are three primary tumors that arise in the testicle: **seminoma, embryonal cell carcinoma,** and **teratocarcinoma.** It is too early in our experience to say whether these have characteristic ultrasound appearances that would permit a specific pathologic diagnosis. It seems, however, that teratocarcinoma and embryonal cell carcinoma are fairly echogenic tumors with multiple areas of both increased and decreased echo production. Seminomas seem to be more homogeneous tumors, considerably less dense than the adjacent testicular tissue. **Lymphoma,** a non-primary tumor that occurs in the testicle, is also an echo-poor lesion and can even be mistaken for a cyst if the sonographer is not wary. The important thing to remember is that neoplasms always vary in texture from the normal gland. For this reason any deviation from a monotonously homogeneous pattern of echoes is very suggestive of cancer.

The exception that proves the rule department: Even though we feel that any focal solid lesion of the testicle should be considered a carcinoma, there are some exceptions. We have already mentioned the irregular testicular pattern in acute orchitis, but this is not usually a diagnostic problem because of the dramatic clinical presentation. Acute testicular hemorrhage from trauma is another source of focal lesions, but again the clinical setting is usually diagnostic. Focal areas of testicular infarction present a more difficult problem. These areas presumably arise from prior infection or trauma and, in their healed stage, appear as very high-intensity echoes, often

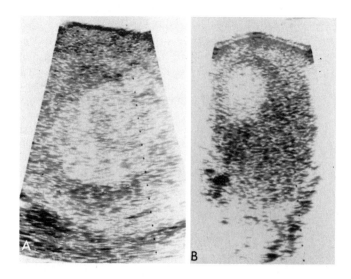

Figure 14–8. Any focal solid lesion in the testicle, regardless of size, should be considered a malignant tumor.

A. A large embryonal cell carcinoma of the testicle.

B. A small seminoma of the testicle.

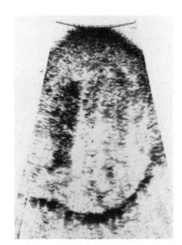

Figure 14–9. Testicular infarction leads to necrosis, fibrosis, and often calcifications. The ultrasonic appearance is one of extreme echo heterogeneity with some areas of acoustic shadowing.

with some calcifications and shadowing (Figure 14–9). It is probably not possible to differentiate such areas from carcinoma on the basis of the ultrasound appearance alone, but usually patients with focal infarctions will have a history of previous testicular trauma or infection. Most testicular tumors arise de novo in a previously normal testicle.

The epididymis can become focally enlarged by acute inflammation (**epididymitis**). This is usually associated with a concomitant orchitis, and the clinical findings are diagnostic.

PERSPECTIVE

We are not being chauvinistic when we say that the scrotum is one of the most satisfying areas of ultrasound diagnosis. It is readily accessible and easily scanned, there are relatively few pathologic conditions, and the ultrasound appearance of most of the pathologic processes is characteristic. It is particularly helpful to be able to say that a testicle is normal. Small spermatoceles or other irregularities of the testicle are frequently found during physical examination. The ability to examine the testicle carefully and exclude any focal mass lesions saves the patient considerable anxiety and may spare him exploratory surgery. On the other side of the coin, tiny carcinomas of the testicle can be identified; these lesions probably would not otherwise be diagnosed until they had grown much larger. It is reasonable to expect that we can favorably alter the long-term prognosis for such patients.

BIBLIOGRAPHY

Leopold, G. R., Woo, V. L., Scheible, W., et al.: High resolution ultrasonography of scrotal pathology. *Radiology 131*:719 (1979).
(A good discussion with excellent illustrations. The scans were performed with a high-resolution machine.)

Arger, P. H., Mulhern, C. B., Jr., Coleman, B. G., et al.: Prospective analysis of the value of scrotal ultrasound. *Radiology 141*:763 (1981).
(A prospective analysis of 69 cases; these authors found ultrasound very accurate.)

Chapter 15

THYROID AND PARATHYROID

High-resolution limited-range scanners have given us an entirely new look at the thyroid and the parathyroid glands. Oddly enough, however, the experience has been different in these two areas. Whereas scanning the thyroid is fraught with uncertainties as to its role in the care of thyroid disease, ultrasound has proved to be a boon to the surgeon dealing with parathyroid problems.

There can be no question that ultrasound provides an unparalleled view of the thyroid gland; both the distribution and the extent of disease are easily and more accurately revealed by this technique than by any other procedure short of pathologic examination. Because masses in the thyroid are so common as patients age, however, locating "disease" in the gland is of only limited usefulness unless there is some way to differentiate potentially lethal from benign change. Herein lies the rub: The ultrasonic appearance of "abnormality" in the thyroid is rarely specific enough to make a definite diagnosis.

The situation is very different with the parathyroids. To date, experience suggests that the ultrasound scanner is accurate in identifying abnormal parathyroids, as long as they are in the neck. The nature of disease in the parathyroids is such that this is useful information for the clinician and aids greatly in treatment.

NORMAL APPEARANCE

Anatomy

There is considerable anatomic variation in the shape and size of the normal thyroid gland. Typically, there are two cylindrical lobes located at either side of the trachea, connected by a thin bridge of tissue, the isthmus (Figure 15–1). The most craniad portions of the right and left lobes (the upper poles) usually are located near the lower portion of the thyroid cartilage (the "Adam's apple"), and the caudad portions (the lower poles) extend for about 5 cm, terminating just above the manubrium. The isthmus connects the lower poles of the two lobes and passes across the top of the trachea. The entire gland lies underneath the thin muscles of the anterior part of the neck and above the carotid arteries and jugular veins.

In addition to the thyroid there are other important anatomic structures in the neck that we want to be sure to recognize. First, there are the common carotid arteries, running craniad from beneath the clavicle. They lie lateral and slightly posterior (dorsal) to the lobes of the thyroid. Slightly further laterally and just anterior (ventral) to the carotid arteries are the internal jugular veins. The veins vary more than the arteries. With normal respiration they may be only barely perceptible, but if you ask the patient to hold his breath and bear down with his stomach muscles (a Valsalva maneuver) you will see them balloon out dramatically. Between the skin and the vessels lie the muscles of the anterior part of the neck, the sternocleidomastoids and the straps. They originate near the midline at the level of the clavicles and run to the base of the skull, creating the V that is obvious in the front of the neck.

The parathyroids are located just beneath (dorsal to) the thyroid; they are, in fact, embedded in the thyroid. There are usually four, one at each pole of the two lobes of the thyroid. In the same region there is a group of structures comprising the longus colli muscle, the inferior thyroidal blood vessels, and the recurrent laryngeal nerve. Together they make up the neurovascular bundle, an important landmark when one is looking for parathyroid enlargement. The normal parathyroids cannot be distinguished from the adjacent thyroid and neurovascular bundle.

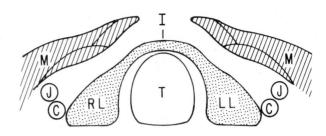

Figure 15–1. The right and left lobes of the thyroid lie between the trachea and the carotid arteries. The small bridge of tissue connecting their lower poles is called the isthmus. RL = right lobe of thyroid, LL = left lobe of thyroid, I = isthmus, T = trachea, J = jugular vein, C = carotid artery, M = muscles of neck.

Size and Texture

So far things have been relatively straightforward. When it comes to defining normal, however, the trouble begins, because there is wide variability in the appearance of the thyroid gland among patients who have no apparent thyroid disease. In fact, the term *normal* is probably not appropriate. Perhaps *typical* or *commonly seen* would be better. Nowhere is this clearer than when we are dealing with thyroid size and texture. Although the "normal" thyroid lobe is said to be about 5 cm in length by 1.5 cm in diameter, this is quite variable, and in many patients one lobe is larger than the other. Also, a thyroid lobe may be cylindrical, spherical, teardrop-shaped, triangular, or just plain lumpy. This variability occurs not only between individual patients but also between the right and left lobes in the same patient. The isthmus may be 5 mm thick or so thin as to be invisible.

In general the texture of the thyroid consists of uniform high-intensity echoes (Figure 15–2). This "normal" appearance, however, is present in only about two thirds of the population; the other third have one or more of the "abnormal" patterns we shall describe. Abnormality increases in frequency as patients age.

SCANNING TECHNIQUE

Our discussions are limited to scanning with a real-time limited-range, or small parts, scanner. The high frequency (7.5 to 10 mHz) of these instruments is necessary to produce the detailed views upon which our present concepts of thyroid disease are based. We used to attempt examination with manual scanners using lower frequency; gross abnormalities were visible, but the subtle changes that we are going to describe were, for the most part, lost.

Performing a thyroid ultrasound scan with a limited-range scanner is simple enough. The gland is located in the lower anterior part of the neck where it is readily accessible to the ultrasound beam. We examine each lobe of the thyroid separately, both transversely and longitudinally. Because the anatomy is more easily recognized in transverse view, we begin in that plane, starting at the upper pole on one side and scanning down through the lobe to the lower pole. We then look at the same lobe longitudinally. Because the field of view of our small parts scanner cannot encompass the whole gland lengthwise, we have to examine first the upper, then the lower portions both medially and laterally. The procedure is then repeated on the opposite lobe. Finally, we examine the

Figure 15–2. The normal thyroid produces homogeneous high-intensity echoes.

A. A transverse scan through the lower pole of the right lobe of the thyroid *(arrow)*. T = trachea (in an acoustic shadow), C = carotid artery, M = strap muscles of the neck.

B. A longitudinal scan through the lower pole of the right lobe of the thyroid (Th). Solid arrow = strap muscles of neck. Open arrow = thyroid vessels (neurovascular bundle). The scale marks for all the illustrations in this chapter are 2.5 mm apart.

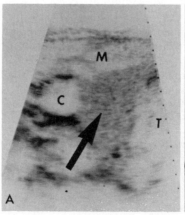
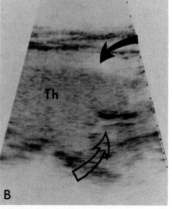

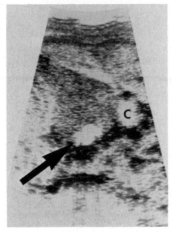

Figure 15–3. Pure cystic lesions of the thyroid are uncommon. This transverse scan through the lower pole of the left lobe demonstrates a 3 mm cyst *(arrow)*. C = carotid artery.

isthmus connecting the lobes. As is our usual practice, we make selected hard copy views to record what we have seen.

PATHOLOGIC APPEARANCE OF THE THYROID

Cystic Masses

Figure 15–3 shows a cyst in the thyroid. Like cystic masses in other organs in the body, it possesses the ultrasonic criteria of a benign cystic process (no internal echoes, smooth posterior wall, and increased sound transmission). Pathologically **thyroid cysts** are areas of homogeneous fluid collection and are not associated with malignant thyroid disease. They may arise from degeneration of **benign solid lesions** of the thyroid. Before the advent of high-resolution ultrasound, it was thought that such cystic lesions of the thyroid were common. We now know that they are relatively **un**common and that most fluid-containing or "cystic" thyroid lesions do not fulfill the ultrasound criteria for a simple cyst but instead contain some solid elements.

Cystic Masses With Solid Elements

Figure 15–4 shows a variety of complex thyroid lesions—cystic lesions with solid elements or, if you prefer, solid lesions with cystic elements. Notice that there is quite a spectrum of such lesions, ranging from those that are nearly cystic to those that are nearly solid. The solid elements of these masses are usually less echogenic than the adjacent thyroid tissue, but they may also contain areas of increased echogenicity or may be identical to the uninvolved tissue. Most of these lesions have a well-defined boundary separating them from the adjacent thyroid tissue; this has been described as a "halo" or "capsule." The most common pathologic diagnosis of these complex thyroid lesions is some type of thyroid **adenoma with cystic degeneration.** The overwhelming majority are benign. Unfortunately, however, **carcinoma** has been occasionally found in such a lesion, so the picture of a cystic mass with solid elements cannot be relied upon as an absolute sign of benign disease.

Solid Masses

Figure 15–5 shows two types of solid masses encountered in the thyroid; both appear as areas of disruption in the high-intensity homogeneity of the thyroid tissue. These solid lesions frequently contain some areas of decreased echo production, but may range widely from total homogeneity to a very heterogeneous appearance and may be made up of high-intensity echoes.

Focal solid lesions often appear to be well demarcated from the surrounding tissue by a "capsule." Intuitively, it would seem that a capsule limiting the mass implies that it is not aggressive and, therefore, not a malignant tumor. This is certainly an attractive hypothesis for the ultrasonographer, and it is true that demonstrating a capsule increases the likelihood that the lesion is benign. Occasionally malignant growths have been found with a capsule, however, so this sign is not absolutely reliable.

Finally, the strength of the echoes within a solid nodule may be an important clue to its nature. If the echoes in the mass are greater than or equal in intensity to those in the normal gland, the probability that the lesion is benign increases. Echoes within cancers are almost always reduced in strength relative to those in the normal gland.

Poorly Defined Masses

Figure 15–6 shows another type of thyroid appearance—the poorly defined, or "permea-

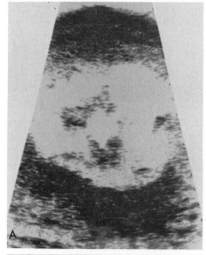
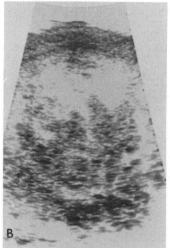
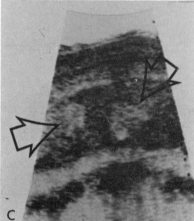

Figure 15–4. Both adenomas and carcinomas of the thyroid have variable appearances ranging from mostly cystic to completely solid.

A. A follicular adenoma that is predominantly cystic with some solid elements.

B. A medullary carcinoma that is predominantly solid with some cystic elements.

C. Two follicular adenomas *(arrows)* that are completely solid.

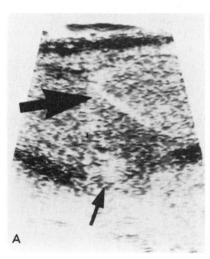
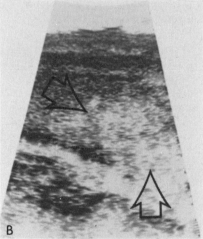

Figure 15–5. The presence of a capsule or "halo" is *not* a reliable sign for differentiating benign from malignant lesions.

A. The two lesions in this gland *(arrows)* were both adenomas, yet one has a well-defined capsule and the other does not.

B. This large, irregularly bounded lesion *(arrows)* was a benign adenoma.

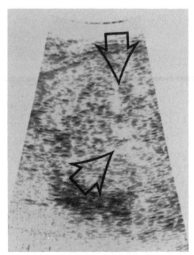

Figure 15–6. Thyroiditis causes the involved portions of the gland to become heterogeneous in texture *(arrows)*. We have also seen this appearance from carcinoma and follicular adenomas.

tive," mass. One might conclude from its appearance that this type of lesion should be a carcinoma; it seems to be growing into the surrounding tissue. In most of the patients we have seen with this finding, however, the pathologic diagnosis has been either **thyroiditis**, some type of **adenoma**, or **nonspecific goiter**. To be fair, some **malignant tumors** of the thyroid (particularly medullary carcinoma) have had this appearance; but more often than not, this poorly defined, permeative pattern has indicated benign disease.

Generalized Enlargement

Whenever a thyroid lobe is increased in size (known clinically as a **goiter**), the ultrasound appearance is usually a combination of one or more of the foregoing. There may be several focal lesions, some with cystic areas and others solid. Some of the focal lesions may have capsules, while others do not. There may even be some regions with poorly defined echo abnormalities. Ultrasonically there is no way to identify malignancy within such a gland.

"DISEASES" OF THE THYROID

So how do we put all this together and come to a sensible diagnosis when we find an abnormality on a thyroid scan? It is not easy. There are many terms that you will find bandied about

in the thyroid literature; let us review the more important of them to see what the ultrasonic appearance might be expected to be.

Goiter

The term *goiter* is not really a pathologic description, but a clinical one. It refers to any enlarged thyroid gland. It is most commonly used to describe a condition of generalized thyroid hyperplasia from hormonal stimulation (which can be induced either by low thyroid output from the gland itself or from a primary abnormality of thyroid stimulating hormone). We have already described the ultrasound appearance of this process—any one or a combination of the various abnormal appearances of the thyroid gland.

Multinodular Goiter

This is also a clinical term and is usually applied to an enlarged thyroid gland that has multiple palpable nodules. These patients usually have radionuclide scans showing focal areas of decreased thyroid activity and may or may not have clinical thyroid abnormalities. The ultrasound appearance of the multinodular goiter is one of multiple focal thyroid lesions. The entire spectrum from cystic to solid may be represented, and capsules may be present. When these lesions are examined under the microscope, the pathologist usually labels them as some type of thyroid adenoma. Although carcinoma can occur in the multinodular goiter, its incidence is probably no greater than in the patient with no thyroid masses. Obviously, a carcinoma will be very difficult to identify in the multinodular goiter patient.

Benign Tumor (Adenoma)

Pathologists consider a thyroid mass that does not metastasize to distant sites or show aggressive infiltrative behavior to be an adenoma. (There are several different types of adenoma, which need not concern us as ultrasonologists). As we have seen, adenomas are very common in the thyroid gland, increasingly so with age. Here again, the appearance can vary from a solid mass with echoes greater in intensity than the normal gland to what appears to be a "pure" cyst.

Carcinoma

As we have stated already, cancers have reduced echogenicity, but they may also have other signs usually associated with benign disease (capsule, cysts), so it is never possible to exclude carcinoma absolutely. Pathologists recognize four different types of carcinoma on the basis of the appearance of the abnormal cells under the microscope. These different types of malignant growth vary in aggressiveness; some such as the anaplastic type almost always cause death, while others such as the follicular and papillary types are very nonaggressive and barely affect the patient at all. Pathologists themselves say that it can be difficult to decide whether a papillary or follicular lesion is an adenoma or a carcinoma. To complicate matters further, the majority of thyroid "carcinomas" are of these types.

Applied imprecision department: The implications of this diagnostic uncertainty can be profound, particularly for the lay public. You may recall that in the past there has been considerable concern that previous irradiation of the thyroid gland increases the incidence of thyroid cancer. Much public attention was focused on this fact, and many millions of dollars were spent in an attempt to find all persons who had previously been exposed to radiation in order to evaluate them for thyroid cancer. This whole project is now shrouded in controversy. First, the "cancers" that were found in these patients were mostly the follicular or papillary type that do not generally pose a significant long-term threat to the patient. Moreover, it has subsequently been found that there probably was not a real increase in carcinoma in irradiated patients; the apparent increase was due simply to the fact that the thyroid gland was more carefully examined in these patients than in the general public, and therefore, more subtle lesions were discovered. When the same strict examination criteria were applied to control groups who did not receive radiation, a similar incidence of new tumors was discovered. All of this work was done before the development of the high-resolution ultrasound scanner. If such a group of patients were examined by modern ultrasound, it is almost certain that even more tumors would be found in both groups. The unanswered question is what to do about these "tumors" inasmuch as it remains to be shown that they pose a threat to the patient's life.

Thyroiditis

Thyroiditis is the fairly straightforward clinical diagnosis of a condition in which the thyroid gland is somewhat enlarged and usually tender. There are also associated endocrine abnormalities. Imaging procedures are usually not performed in these patients. The patients we have examined generally show a diffuse increase in heterogeneity with areas of poorly defined, permeative patterns of reduced echo intensity.

PERSPECTIVE

Although the present state of knowledge about the ultrasound diagnosis of disease in the thyroid is somewhat discouraging, we must not lose heart. The problem is not that ultrasound is no good; rather it is too good and provides us with more information than we know how to use. At present, the greatest promise seems to be in combining ultrasound with fine needle aspiration biopsy. Lesions can be localized precisely, and *all* suspicious areas, *not just those palpable or discernible by radionuclide scan*, can be examined. Also, it seems that some types of lesions can be classified as benign, viz., (1) pure cysts and (2) solid lesions with a capsule and echo intensities equal to or greater than the normal gland.

The concept of the "solitary nodule" upon which many of the principles of contemporary thyroid care are based must be questioned. It has been demonstrated that single thyroid nodules are much rarer than was assumed when the only means of thyroid evaluation was by physical examination or radionuclide scan, and there is no guarantee that one or more of the multiple lesions will not be malignant.

People who live in glass houses department: Do not let your clinical colleagues harass you because of your inability to make specific diagnoses in the thyroid. The ultrasound criteria may not yet be well defined, but they hold greater promise for defining disease in the thyroid than anything else available. Clinical examination and palpation are known to be unreliable; even a skilled clinician can palpate less than half the focal lesions present in the thyroid. Radionuclide imaging is no better. We have found that many of the lesions seen on ultrasound cannot be visualized with state-of-the-art radioisotope scanning. In fact, the insensitivity of the previous "gold standard" led to an inappropriate diagnostic algorithm—the "solitary" thyroid nodule. Patients who were previously felt to have solitary thyroid nodules underwent a long diagnostic procedure to evaluate these lesions. We now know that at least one-third of these so-called solitary nodules are actually multiple, and spending so much effort to chase down any one of them while ignoring the others has to be questioned.

PATHOLOGIC APPEARANCE OF THE PARATHYROIDS

All clinically important disease of the parathyroids involves abnormality of calcium metabolism because of increased parathormone production. The treatment is surgical removal of the abnormal gland. The tumors are usually small, however, and can be located anywhere in the neck or mediastinum, so it has been difficult in the past for the surgeon to know where to go hunting for them. Ultrasound has proved to be valuable in this situation. Examination of the parathyroids is similar to that of the adrenals in that the *normal parathyroid glands are too small and have an echo texture too much like the thyroid to be clearly identified, even with high-resolution scanners.*

The pathologic processes involved here are **hyperplasia, adenoma,** and **carcinoma.** All produce similar ultrasonic pictures; they enlarge the gland into easily recognizable, relatively echo-free masses dorsal to the thyroid (Figure 15–7). Differentiation as to specific diagnosis is not necessary. If a parathyroid can be recognized, it is abnormal, and surgical removal is appropriate. When a patient is suspected of having a parathyroid mass because of clinical findings (elevated serum calcium or serum para-

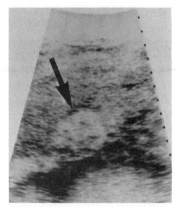

Figure 15–7. If a parathyroid gland can be easily seen *(arrow)*, it is abnormal. This lesion was a parathyroid adenoma.

thormone levels or both), an ultrasound examination should be performed to see whether the mass can be found in the neck. If an enlarged parathyroid can be identified, it will almost always lie near the thyroid. Occasionally the involved gland is located either in the mediastinum, behind the trachea, or near the angle of the jaw. In these cases, ultrasound will not be helpful except to show that the mass is *not* near the thyroid; some other diagnostic method (angiography or computed tomography) will have to be undertaken for localization. It is important also to realize that more than one parathyroid might be abnormal; for this reason a thorough scan of the thyroid area on both sides of the trachea should always be performed.

BIBLIOGRAPHY

Scheible, W., Leopold, G., Woo, V., et al.: High resolution real-time ultrasonography of thyroid nodules. *Radiology 133:*413 (1979).
(This is the first description of the new ball game of high-resolution thyroid ultrasound. The authors show that palpation and radionuclide scans miss lots of lesions.)

Herle, A. J. V., Rich, P., Britt-Morie, E., et al.: The thyroid nodule. *American Journal of Internal Medicine 96:*221 (1982).
(An excellent discussion of the problems in evaluating thyroid disease. The data considered do not include high-resolution ultrasound, and hence the authors overestimate the prevalence of the "solitary" nodule.)

Simeone, J. F., Mueller, P. R., Ferrucci, J. T., Jr., et al.: High resolution real-time sonography of the parathyroid. *Radiology 141:*745 (1981).
(An excellent discussion of parathyroid ultrasound: all you need to know.)

Chapter 16

MISCELLANEOUS EXAMINATIONS

When assembling any text that covers a field as broad as ultrasound, there are inevitably a few topics that are hard to work in. They do not merit an individual chapter, either because there is too little to say about them or because they are too new to have established a definitive role. We will discuss a potpourri of such topics in this final chapter.

Chest

Ultrasound of the chest is straightforward. Normally there is little we have to offer because in the normal chest air-filled lungs repel the sound beam. And, if this were not enough, the area is obscured by the ribs as well. When air in the lung is replaced by fluid or solid tissue, however, ultrasound can make pictures of it. Occasionally we are called on to help sort out the cause of an opacity in the thorax and to decide whether it represents fluid or solid tissue.

We have found it easiest to scan the chest with the patient sitting upright and leaning over the back of a chair or an over-bed table. The ultrasound scanner is then oriented along the intercostal spaces of the back so as to avoid the ribs. It is always helpful to have a recent chest film at hand so you know where to look.

In what situations might ultrasound scanning be useful? First, we can tell whether the chest under the ultrasound beam contains normal air-filled lung or whether this has been replaced by soft tissue. The normal air-filled lung will reflect the ultrasound beam completely, and we will see nothing on our scan except reverberation artifact (Figure 16–1). Fluid or solid tissue, on the other hand, will allow the beam to penetrate and produce an image. Second, we can say whether the aerated lung has been replaced by fluid or solid tissue; we use the same criteria as in the abdomen for making this distinction. Figure 16–2 shows a pleural effusion

with a small tab of collapsed lung floating within it. Generally, fluid will be echo-free, while consolidation will contain echoes of varying intensity. Occasionally, debris floating within pleural fluid will produce echoes and create confusion; in our experience, however, this has not been a common problem. Finally, we can localize effusions to aid in aspiration. Here we would urge you to have the aspiration performed without moving the patient, especially if only a small volume of fluid is present.

Superficial Masses

Any lumps or bumps that are palpable in the superficial tissues in any part of the body are fair game for ultrasound examination. As in the chest, the major information to be gained is whether the mass is solid or fluid-containing. The development of the limited-range high-resolution scanner has greatly facilitated the examination of superficial masses, and with one of these machines the examination is almost trivial. All that is required is to place the scanner over the suspicious area and move it back and forth so that you can have a look at the entire lesion. It is no trick to say whether the lesion is solid or cystic and whether or not it is connected to any blood vessels. The only hazard in this area is failure to remember that lymph nodes often appear cystic. Before you call any superficial lump cystic, be certain to check for the presence of a smooth back wall and enhanced sound transmission, and always include the possibility of an enlarged lymph node in your differential diagnosis.

Figure 16–3 is an example of a superficial scan of the radial artery and demonstrates an aneurysm of this vessel. Figure 16–4 is a scan of a mass on the back of the leg, showing a fluid-filled cyst dissecting into the soft tissues— a Baker's cyst of the knee. We could show many other examples of isolated lumps and bumps and give their diagnoses, but you get the idea.

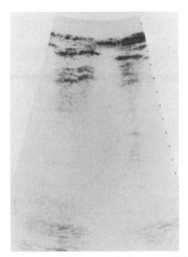

Figure 16–1. In the normal chest, air-filled lung totally reflects the sound beam and the scan shows only acoustic shadowing and reverberations.

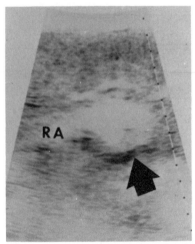

Figure 16–3. Aneurysms of superficial arteries are easily identified. This scan of a pulsatile "lump" on the wrist demonstrates a radial artery aneurysm *(arrow)*. RA = radial artery. Scale marks are 2.5 mm apart.

Isolate the suspicious mass, examine it thoroughly with your scanner, decide whether it is solid or cystic, and finally describe its relation to any surrounding vessels.

Carotid Artery

There is considerable interest in using ultrasound to evaluate the carotid arteries. The number of potential patients is staggering when one considers that as many as 30 million Americans suffer from clinically significant atherosclerotic disease of these vessels. At present there is only one good method for evaluating the carotid arteries—arteriography. Unfortunately, this procedure is expensive and complicated and carries a significant morbidity and even a small risk of death. It is not suitable for use as a screening procedure for the vast num-

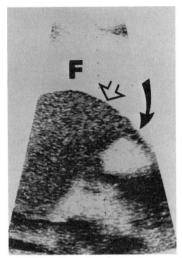

Figure 16–2. When the thorax is opacified, the ultrasound scan can distinguish fluid from solid tissue. This intercostal scan shows a large pleural effusion (F). There are consolidation in the underlying lung *(open arrow)* and adhesions to the diaphragm *(curved arrow)*.

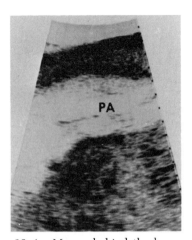

Figure 16–4. Masses behind the knee are com mon. This longitudinal scan through a popliteal mass shows it to be partially fluid-filled and separate from the popliteal artery (PA). This is a common popliteal cyst, or Baker's cyst.

ber of potential patients. Many indirect means of studying the carotid artery have been used in the past 20 years, including various forms of carotid bruit analysis, Doppler spectral flow analysis, directional Doppler detection of internal and external carotid flow, pulse analysis of the internal carotid system, Doppler imaging, and thermography. Although many of these methods have enthusiastic supporters, none has established itself as a reproducible and reliable clinical tool. The high-resolution, limited-range, real-time ultrasound scanners were primarily designed as a means of studying the carotid arteries.

If you are going to perform carotid artery examinations, you must have one of these special purpose units. Conventional scanners, even using a high-frequency transducer, do not have good enough resolution to resolve the small, sub-millimeter sized ulcers that are harbingers of significant disease. It is true that you can make pictures of the carotid artery and identify gross atherosclerotic plaques with conventional scanners, but this type of information is not really adequate for clinical purposes.

We scan the carotid arteries with the patient lying supine, but with the shoulder of the side being examined elevated on a pillow. The head is turned to the opposite side, and the carotid artery is scanned both longitudinally and in cross-section from the level of the clavicle until it vanishes beneath the angle of the mandible. Longitudinal scans are the easiest to perform and give the most satisfying views of the common carotid artery and its bifurcation into internal and external carotid branches (Figure 16–5). While longitudinal scans are valuable for getting the "lay of the land," they are not adequate for diagnosis. Remember, the scan plane of these limited-range scanners is very thin, and a single longitudinal view samples only a thin sliver of the vessels; disease slightly off-axis can be easily overlooked and underestimated. It is, therefore, necessary to study the artery with transverse scans in order to evaluate the severity of atherosclerotic disease accurately.

The ultrasonographer is trying to determine two things: how much the lumen of the common or internal carotid artery is compromised by atherosclerotic plaques and whether there are any ulcerations within the plaques. It is of little value to determine only that atherosclerotic plaques are present; virtually all patients over 50 years of age or with any kind of symptoms will have plaques in the arteries. What is necessary is to decide whether these plaques are

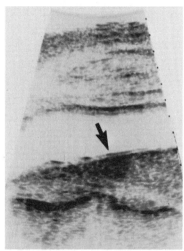

Figure 16–5. The endothelium of the normal carotid artery is thin and smooth (arrow). This is a longitudinal scan of the common carotid artery just proximal to its bifurcation. Scale marks are 2.5 mm apart.

significant enough to be causing clinical problems and need further evaluation or treatment.

Figure 16–6 shows two types of atherosclerotic plaques. "Soft" plaque is defined as an atherosclerotic lesion that does not contain calcium and does not cast an acoustic shadow. "Hard" plaque contains calcium and causes well-defined acoustic shadowing. Figure 16–7 illustrates both significant and insignificant reduction of the carotid artery lumen. There is some controversy as to what constitutes a "significant" lesion. Everyone agrees that if the lumen area is not reduced by 50 per cent or more, the lesion is insignificant. Lumen reductions of between 50 and 70 per cent are considered a "gray" zone. Between 70 and 90 per cent lumen reduction is probably significant, and greater than 90 per cent reduction is definitely significant.

Figure 16–8 shows an ulcer in an atherosclerotic plaque. The presence of an ulcer is considered clinically significant, because ulcers are felt to be the source of small blood clots or emboli. Over 80 per cent of strokes are due to such emboli.

Because ultrasound scanning of the carotid artery is so new, its ultimate value is not known. We have been performing this procedure for nearly two years and correlating all of our results with our arteriography. We have found that, *when the vessel is well seen*, ultrasound is as accurate as arteriography in detecting the degree of plaque formation and compromise of

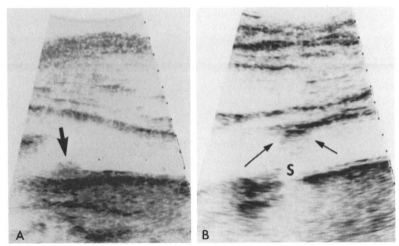

Figure 16–6. Atherosclerotic plaque is either "soft," meaning it does not contain calcium, or "hard," when calcium is present.

A. A longitudinal scan at the bifurcation of the carotid artery showing "soft" plaque *(arrow)*.

B. "Hard" plaque *(arrows)* on the anterior wall of the common carotid artery. The calcium in the plaque causes shadowing (S), which obscures the back wall of the vessel. Scale marks are 2.5 mm apart.

the lumen. Our early success in detecting ulcers was limited, but since we have been using more aggressive criteria for making this diagnosis, we have had accuracy comparable to that of the arteriogram in this area as well. In diagnosing an ulcer ultrasonically one must be very aggressive; any irregularity in the surface of the plaque should be considered an ulcer until proved otherwise.

There is a Catch-22, however. Ultrasound results are only good when the arteries can be well seen, and this occurs in only 50 per cent of patients. The problem is a familiar one: acoustic shadowing. Many plaques contain cal-

cium and cast acoustic shadows, as illustrated in Figure 16–6B. When such plaques are located on the anterior wall of the vessel, the shadow hides the posterior wall from our view. Then we cannot tell whether there is any posterior wall present, let alone get an estimate of the amount of luminal narrowing or evaluate ulcers. From our early experience it would appear that high-resolution ultrasound evaluation of the carotid arteries may be very useful for a group of patients in whom the artery is well seen. Those patients in whom ultrasound is not adequate will need to have thorough evaluation by another method.

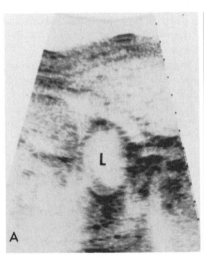 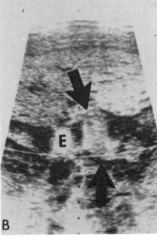

Figure 16–7. Arterial lumen reduction should be evaluated on *transverse* rather than longitudinal scans.

A. Transverse section of the common carotid artery just proximal to the bifurcation. There is some plaque, but the lumen (L) is not significantly narrowed.

B. A transverse scan just above the bifurcation of the carotid artery. The external carotid (E) is normal, but extensive plaque has reduced the lumen of the internal carotid *(arrows)* to a pinpoint. Scale marks are 2.5 mm apart.

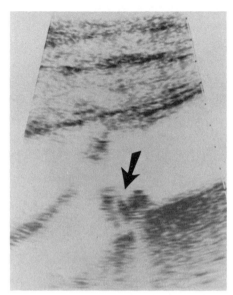

Figure 16–8. Any irregularities in the surface of a plaque indicate ulceration *(arrow)*. Scale marks are 2.5 mm apart.

Breast

There is even more interest in ultrasound scanning of the breast than in scanning of the carotid artery. The reasons are well known. One of every sixteen American women will develop breast cancer in her lifetime; the odds worsen to one of six when risk factors are present. There are approximately 70 million women in this country old enough to be at risk for breast cancer. The current methods of early detection of breast cancer are not good; the most sensitive, x-ray mammography, fails to detect as many as 30 per cent of early cancers. Physical examination and other methods have proved even less accurate. Finally, there is concern by some people that repeated x-ray mammography may actually place a woman at higher risk for developing cancer.

It is little wonder, then, that much effort and expense is being devoted to developing an ultrasound scanner that might be capable of improving on the performance of x-ray mammography. It has become clear that conventional ultrasound scanners are of no value; all they are able to do is tell whether a palpable lesion is cystic or solid, and this is not very useful information. (A palpable lesion can easily be aspirated with a needle to determine whether it is cystic; if not, it can be removed.) There is not much value in having another method of characterizing a lesion that has al-ready been detected; rather, what is needed is a better way of finding tiny breast cancers before they are too large to be treatable.

At present there are several specially designed breast scanners commercially available. The clinical experience with these machines is limited, and the early results are not particularly encouraging. While these scanners seem to be nearly as good as x-ray mammography in classifying general breast disease (such as fibrocystic disease) or normality, they have not yet been shown to be of value in attacking the main problem, detection of minimal lesions. There is some suggestion that in skilled and dedicated hands, these instruments may be as valuable as x-ray mammography; and inasmuch as they do not involve radiation, there may be some role for them in the future. The field is too new and the results are too sketchy to draw any conclusions at this time. We do not believe that the average clinical ultrasonographer should be involved in breast scanning at present.

Neonatal Brain

Ultrasound examination of the neonatal brain is an exciting new field. Any of the latest generation of real-time scanners is capable of making excellent images of the brain in infants of less than three months of age. After that, the skull thickens to the point at which most of the acoustic windows are lost.

We examine the skull in both coronal and sagittal planes and begin coronally because orientation is easier. Fortunately, the transducers of most real-time scanners are small and can even fit into incubators or Isolettes for examination of infants in the nursery. Unless the baby is very small, it will be necessary to scan through the anterior fontanelle; otherwise there will be too much attenuation by the bone in the skull. We almost always use this acoustic window because we find that it is convenient and allows ready anatomic orientation. Sagittal scans through the anterior fontanelle are also very helpful. We scan in that direction routinely after we have done the coronal views. Figure 16–9 shows the position of the scan planes we employ.

In our experience the most useful views are the coronal section, which passes from the anterior fontanelle through the basal ganglia (coronal "M"), and the sagittal sections through the lateral ventricle. Figure 16–10A shows a normal coronal "M" section in a premature

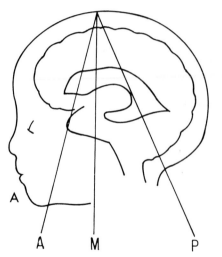
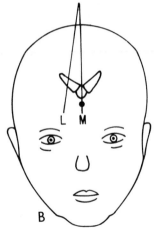

Figure 16–9. A. Lateral view of skull showing the three standard planes for coronal scans through the anterior fontanelle. A = anterior, M = middle, P = posterior.

B. Frontal view of skull showing the standard planes for sagittal sections. M = midline, L = lateral.

baby. The cavum septi pellucidi is readily apparent, but the lateral ventricles should be mere slits—no more than 0.5 mm across. The tissue immediately beneath the lateral ventricles (the germinal matrix) should have the same echo intensity as the tissue above the ventricle (the corpus callosum). Figure 16–10B shows a normal sagittal section through the lateral ventricle in a premature baby. Again, the diameter of the ventricle should be less than 0.5 mm, and the echo intensity of the germinal matrix should be the same as that of the corpus callosum. The choroid plexus of the lateral ventricle appears as an elongated structure of high echo intensity. Some ultrasonologists believe that the choroid is always smooth and any "lumpiness" represents hemorrhage. We have not found this to be the case in our patients;

the choroid can be lumpy even in the absence of bleeding.

There are two intracranial conditions that commonly afflict premature infants: hemorrhage and hydrocephalus.

Intracranial hemorrhage is very common in premature infants for reasons that are not entirely understood. The hemorrhage usually arises in the germinal matrix and may remain confined there or spread to involve other areas of the brain, even the ventricles and the subarachnoid space itself. Hemorrhage first appears on the scan as increased echogenicity immediately beneath the lateral ventricles. Figure 16–11 shows examples of minimal and severe intracranial hemorrhage.

Hydrocephalus is usually a complication of prior intracranial hemorrhage. The normal cer-

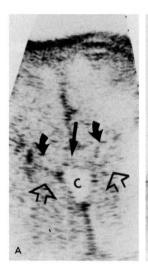
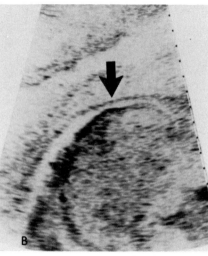

Figure 16–10. The lateral ventricles are very small in normal infants.

A. This is a normal midcoronal scan showing the prominent cavum septi pellucidi (C), and the tiny lateral ventricles *(curved arrows)*. The echogenicity of the tissue just beneath the lateral ventricles *(open arrows)*—the germinal matrix and basal ganglia—should *not* be greater than that of the tissue above the cavum *(straight arrow)*—the corpus callosum.

B. A sagittal section through a normal lateral ventricle *(arrow)*. The choroid plexus is the thin, irregular band of intense echoes on the floor of the ventricle. Scale marks are 2.5 mm apart.

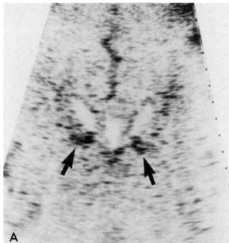

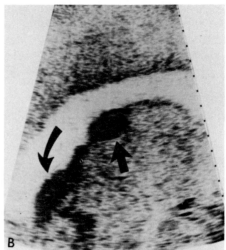

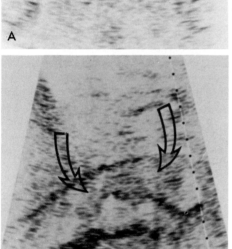

Figure 16–11. Intracranial hemorrhage begins in the germinal matrix and may or may not spread into the choroid plexus and ventricles. It is always associated with hydrocephalus, and the severity of the ventricular dilatation is usually proportional to the extent of the bleeding.

A. Minimal bilateral germinal matrix hemorrhage *(arrows)* and hydrocephalus seen on coronal scan. Hemorrhage causes the echogenicity of the germinal matrix to exceed that of the corpus callosum.

B. More severe hemorrhage and hydrocephalus are shown in this sagittal scar through a lateral ventricle. The hemorrhage originated in the germinal matrix *(straight arrow)*, but may have dissected into the choroid plexus, causing it to enlarge *(curved arrow)*.

C. This sagittal section shows a lateral ventricle filled with blood clot and distended *(open arrows)*. The origin of the hemorrhage was the germinal matrix *(solid arrow)*. Scale marks are 2.5 mm apart.

ebral spinal fluid pathways become blocked, usually by edema in the region of the foramen of Monro or by adhesions from intracranial blood. The normal cerebral ventricles are nearly collapsed in newborn infants and are difficult to identify with certainty on the scans. If you can see the cerebral ventricles clearly and if the diameter of the lateral ventricles in either coronal or sagittal views is greater than 0.5 mm, you are dealing with a case of hydrocephalus (see Figure 16–11).

The complete anatomy and scanning techniques for neonatal cerebral ultrasound are beyond the scope of this book. If you are likely to get referrals for this type of scanning, you should consult the reference in the bibliography for further details.

VALEDICTORY

Well, if you have made it this far, you will not have Bartrum and Crow to kick around anymore! We have tried to give you a basic foundation in ultrasound. You should be ready to go out, take transducer in hand, and begin making diagnoses. It is important that you also read what others have written in the field; as everyone knows, there is more than one way to scan a cat!* At a minimum you should look into the bibliography at the end of each of the chapters. It is also important to keep abreast of the newest publications; ultrasound is a rapidly

---

*Courtesy of H. Z. Mellins, M.D.

changing field. We have tried to convey our experience and some of the (often painful) lessons we have learned in our laboratory. We hope that if you have read and understood our message, you will have a firm foundation on which to build your own ultrasound expertise.

BIBLIOGRAPHY

Cole-Beuglet, C., Goldberg, B. B., Kurtz, A. B., et al.: Ultrasound mammography: a comparison with radiographic mammography. *Radiology 139*:693 (1981).
(This is the only *good* article on ultrasound and the breast.)

Doust, B. D., Baum, J. K., Maklad, N. F., et al.: Ultrasonic evaluation of pleural opacities. *Radiology 114*:135 (1975).
(Although this article is old, it is among the best on the subject of chest ultrasound. There is nothing much new.)

Wolson, A. H., Kaupp, H. A., and McDonald, K.: Ultrasound of arterial graft surgery complications. *American Journal of Roentgenology 133*:869 (1979).
(A good discussion of a common clinical problem, this paper has nice illustrations of peripheral artery aneurysms and other masses.)

Sauerbrei, E. E., Digney, M., Harrison, P. B., et al.: Ultrasonic evaluation of neonatal intracranial hemorrhage and its complications. *Radiology 139*:677 (1981).
(There are numerous articles and even a book on this subject. We believe this is the best study and the place to begin your reading.)

INDEX

Italic numbers in this index refer to illustrations.

Cyst(s) (*Continued*)
  hepatic, 94, *95*
  ovarian, physiologic, 131, *131*, 133
  pancreatic, 116, *117*
  renal parenchymal, 122, *123*, *124*
  scrotal, 159, *159*, *160*
  theca lutein, 137, *137*
  thyroid, 164, *164*, *165*
Cystadenoma, ovarian, 133, *133*
Cystic duct, 98, *99*
Cystitis, 139

D/A converter, 34
Damping, axial resolution and, 14
Decibel, 4
Defects, anatomic, fetal, 150
Demodulation, 25
Density, picture, gain and, 60
  tissue, attenuation and, 4
  impedance and, 5
Dermoid, ovarian, 133, *134*
Detection, 25
Diabetes mellitus, nephropathy in, 121, *122*
  polyhydramnios and, 153
Differentiation, 25
Diffraction, 5
Digital memory storage system, 25, 31–33, *33*
Discs, as hard copy, 62
  floppy, 33, 35
Dissecting aneurysm, aortic, 86
Distortion, in oscilloscope display, 33
  in video display, 34
Dorsal, definition of, 74
"Doughnut appearance," in lymph node metastasis, 88, *88*
"Down-the-tail" view of pancreas, 112, *113*, *114*
Ducts, bile. See *Bile ducts.*
  pancreatic, normal, 109, *109*
   pathologic appearance of, 115, *116*
Duodenum, air in, artifacts from, 38
   gallstone obstruction and, 140
  atresia of, fetal, 153
Duplication, of kidney, partial, 120, *121*
  of uterus, 130
Dynamic range, digital memory and, 32
  in video display, 34

Echo, principle of, 1
  production of, 5
  quantification of, 25
Echogenic bile, 101, *102*
Ectopic pregnancy, 133, 136, 137
"Electric toothbrush" scanning method, 28, *28*, *29*
Electronic calipers, 32, 34
"Electronic lens," of phased-array transducer, 19, *19*
Electronic noise, artifacts from, 48
Electronic real time, 29, *30*
Embryonal cell carcinoma, testicular, 160, *160*
Encephalocele, fetal, 153
Endometrioma, 133
Endometritis, 132
Endometrium, carcinoma of, 132
  echoes from, 130, *130*
Enhancement, artifacts from, 39, *40*
   simulating metastasis, 47, *49*
  renal cysts and, 122

Epididymis, normal, 156, *157*
  spermatocele of, 159, *159*
Epididymitis, 161
Examination, obstetrical, reporting of, 154, *154*
  organ-oriented, 65–70, *67–71*
   interpretation of, 70–72
  picture-oriented, 63–65, *64*
Examination room, preparation of, 51
"Excessive bowel gas," body habitus and, 50
Expansion (zoom), control for, 61
"Extra-renal pelvis," 125, *125*

Fallopian tube(s), abscess of, *134*
  normal, 129
Fasting, for gallbladder scan, 99
Fat, artifacts from, 49
  in liver, 93
  in normal pancreas, 108, *109*, 115
Female pelvis, normal, 129–131, *130*, *131*
  sector scan of, *54*
Fetal lobulations, of kidney, 119
Fetus(es), age of, 134, 135, 146–149, *147*, 148 (table)
  growth retardation of, 152
  number of, 140, 142
  presentation of, 140–142, *141*
  size of, 140
  viability of, 136
  weight of, 153
  well-being of, 140, 149–152, *150*, *151*
Fibroid(s), uterine, 132, *132*, 134, *134*
  in pregnancy, 146, *146*
Fibrolipomatosis, of renal sinus, 124, *124*
Fibrosis, retroperitoneal, 88, 127
Film, as hard copy, 62
Fixed-focus transducers, 17, *17*, 29
Floppy discs, information storage on, 33
Focal contraction, of uterine wall, 146, *146*
Focal length, transducer, 17
Focal zone, transducer, 17
  for general-scanning, 21
Focus, transducer, 17, *17–19*
  artifacts and, 47, *48*, *49*
  fixed, 17, 29
Follicular adenoma, thyroid, *165*
Follicular cysts, ovarian, 131, *131*, 133
Fontanelle, anterior, as acoustic window, 173, *174*
Fracture, pelvic, hematoma from, 88
Frequency, 3, *3*
  attenuation and, *13*
  of transducer, 10, *11*
   bandwidth and, 12, *12*
   gain adjustment and, 60
Fundus, of uterus, 129

Gain, 24, 60, *60*
  adjustment of, for liver scan, 92
  reverberation artifacts and, 43, 46
  time compensated, 23–25, *23*
   adjustment of, 59, *59*
Gallbladder, abdominal anatomy and, 75, *75*
  artifacts in, 44, *46*
  as specular reflector, 7
  in organ-oriented examination, 69, *69*
  nonvisualized, 102, *103*
  normal, 98, *99*